I Promise
to Put My Lipstick
on When I Get There

I Promise to Put My Lipstick on When I Get There:

The Complete Red-Carpet Guide to Staying Gorgeous Through Your Cancer Treatment

by
Kim and Mike Becker

I PROMISE TO PUT MY LIPSTICK ON WHEN I GET THERE

Copyright © 2014 by Kim and Mike Becker
All rights reserved. No part of this book may be used or reproduced in any manner whatsoever without the written permission of the publisher.

10 9 8 7 6 5 4 3 2

ISBN: 978-0-9912451-7-8

Published by
CORBY BOOKS
A Division of Corby Publishing, LP
P.O. Box 93
Notre Dame, IN 46556

Manufactured in the United States of America

This book is dedicated to God, for giving us this amazing project that we, alone, could never have thought up or moved forward. We give all the glory to Him.

To our 12-year-old son, Seth Michael, for his patience, enthusiasm and for giving us our first dollar for this project from his own money when he was four. You are the greatest kid that ever lived.

This book is dedicated to every woman who has battled this ugly disease and showed it that she is boss, that she refused to give in and remained Gorgeous inside and out. That is our true inspiration. You have given more to us than we will ever be able to give to you.

And to the salon owners and stylists who work selflessly every month bringing the Hello Gorgeous! Experience to these women battling cancer, in their own communities, across the United States, through our Affiliate Salon program.

This book is dedicated to you. May all of you win your battle, find your path, and live happy and healthy to 90 years old.

And may the last words you hear be "Hello, Gorgeous!"

About Our Cover Girl

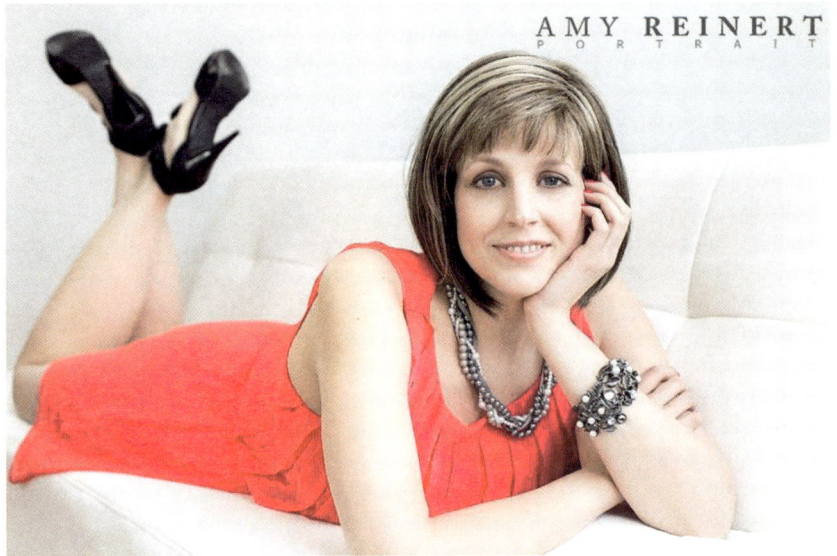

If you can believe it, our beautiful cover girl Kendelle was battling cancer for the second time during the photo shoot for this book. Her vivacious spirit is contagious and we wanted to share her story with you.

It can be found in Chapter 14: Inspirational Stories. Thank you, Kendelle.

Bio, Executive Team and Cover Picture by
   Amy Reinert Photography
Cover Art by Elissa Schmidt
Makeup by Erica Morris
Video Production and Editing by Jeremy Stroup

Testimonials about the Hello Gorgeous! Makeover:

"What a wonderful Day! This is the best day I have had, except for the day I was told I was in remission. Thank you so much."
– Kay

"Words cannot describe how I feel today. An experience of a lifetime! You were outstanding! Bless you and all you do. I will remember this always." – Linda

"All I can say is you've made me feel like me again!! I can't thank you enough!!" – Shelly

"Just when I was feeling that everyone had forgotten about my struggle, you all gave me a whole new attitude. Thank you."
– Jackie

"Thank you so much! You've made me feel beautiful again! AMAZING DAY!!!" – Kathy L.

"HELLO! Thank you for helping me to feel special, beautiful and loved—which is a reflection of you and the life-giving family, friends and people that you have surrounded yourself with to do these Gorgeous makeovers!!
– Elise

"This has been an outstanding day! I would have never thought to do this for myself. I feel great now. Thank you."
— Barb

"Get up even when you don't feel like it! Thank you, Hello Gorgeous!!"
— Cheryl

"Thank you for the wonderful experience. What a way to celebrate life! Never stop living..."
— Kathy

"Throughout this year, I have thought of you often and the wonderful day that you gave me. Never would I have thought that things done on the outside could effect such a change on the inside. What you do is nothing short of magical!"
— Rose Ann

Our organization has had the pleasure of working with Hello Gorgeous! and their mobile unit for over 7 years. We too are a 501c3 who gives aid to women suffering from cancer. Without hesitation, we give the entire Hello Gorgeous! organization great applause for their tireless, cheerful, heartfelt approach to everything they touch. Their burning passion to bring & provide services, showing great concern for a woman to grow in strength, both physical & mental, gain confidence, is unmatched in our community. Watching the transformation, the "reveal" of a woman who was gifted a makeover, will move anyone to tears of joy just being in that moment with them. Their faith is inspiring and evident in all they do and say. It is a priceless service they do to touch the lives of those who are in need and to those who are fortunate enough to bear witness. We look forward to all that they are to become in the months and years ahead.

God Bless,
Helping Her Heal, Inc., a 501c3
Susan Weaver, Treasurer

Table of Contents

What Exactly Is Hello Gorgeous?	xiii
Foreword	xvii
Introduction	xxix
Ch. 1 The Hello Gorgeous! Experience	1
Ch. 2 Attitude First	9
Ch. 3 Comfortable in Your Own Skin	25
Ch. 4 Can't Touch This…Or Can You?	33
Ch. 5 Nails…Your Second Best Feature	37
Ch. 6 The Balder the Head, the Bigger the Earrings	53
Ch. 7 My Hair Is Gone…Now What?	61
Ch. 8 My Hair Has Stayed, But It's Not the Same	83
Ch. 9 My Hair Grew Back…Now What?	89
Ch. 10 Put Your Best Face Forward	101
Ch. 11 Let's Play Dress-Up	119
Ch. 12 Showing One's True Colors	135
Ch. 13 Celebrate!	141
Ch. 14 Inspirational Stories	147
Ch. 15 Stories from the Affiliates	177
Material Lists	189
Glossary of Terms	191
Works Cited	199

What Exactly Is Hello Gorgeous?

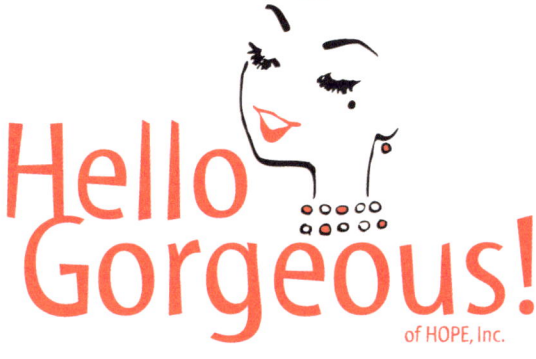

Hello Gorgeous! of HOPE, Inc. is a 501(c)(3) not-for-profit that provides a red-carpet experience for all women battling all cancers, with full spa ambush-style makeovers in one of our 36' mobile DaySpas or by one of our partnering Affiliate Salons across the United States and at no cost to the women.

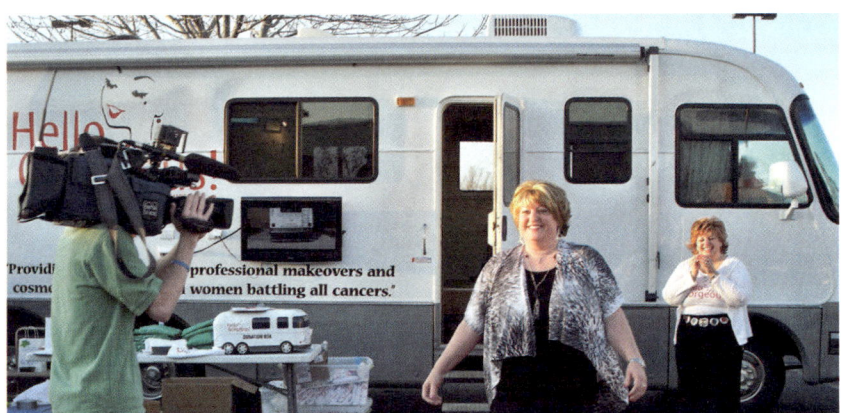

Again, these are surprise makeovers. All women served by our program are nominated by family or friends and their nominations are looked over by a committee, which chooses the women based on merit, need and availability.

Once chosen, arrangements are made with the individual nominating the woman with cancer to have her at a prearranged location or salon for the event. We show up unannounced and:
- Roll out a red carpet
- Surprise them with candy, flowers and a big "Hello, Gorgeous!"
- Treat them to spa services including manicure, pedicure and facial
- Give a hair consultation and makeup application
- Gift them with a new clothing outfit
- And, many times, show off the Gorgeous woman and her "new look" at a prearranged, gathered group of their family and friends called a Reveal.

We have found that the services and education we furnish can allow these women a positive anchor during their battle with cancer; in addition, we provide cosmetic techniques that are education-specific to the effects of their cancer treatments and the side-effects of those treatments. We pamper them for a day and instruct them on how to help conceal the physical damages to their looks with specialized products and techniques that we supply.

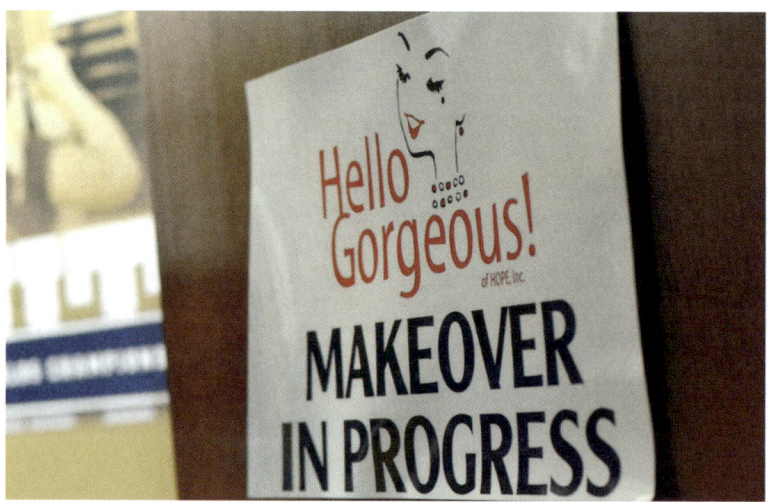

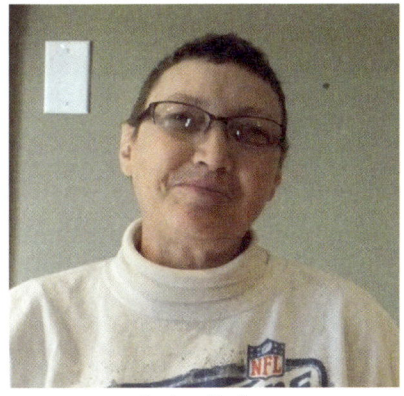 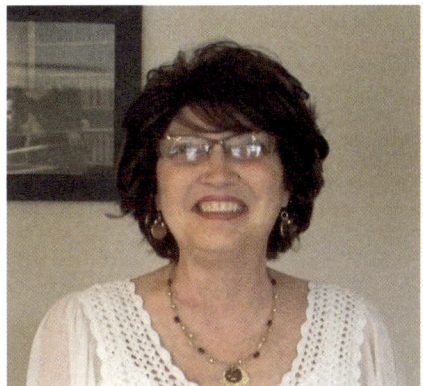

Anita Before	Anita After

Simply stated, our mission is to provide cosmetic aid and education to those battling cancer. It will work to strengthen the knowledge of cancer patients and survivors concerning their hair styling, hair substitution, skincare and cosmetic techniques that will allow them to return to their jobs, their families, their friends and to the general public eye with confidence and courage. We want to help them step back out into the world with some of that confidence and poise taken from them by the disease that they struggle to conquer.

This is the mission and passion of Hello Gorgeous! of HOPE, Inc.

Foreword

I personally can relate to the emotional, psychological and physical trauma that comes from a cancer diagnosis. My mother was only 49 years old when she died from lung cancer. She had never smoked, and before that time had been, overall, a very healthy woman. She survived only nine months after her diagnosis. I can recall watching her deteriorate and fearing the process as well as the outcome. I was only 23 years old and had a younger brother and an older sister. I can recall waiting for help to arrive in the hospital, but it never did. The only "support" I can recall is a person handing us brochures on death and grief during one of our mother's hospital admissions.

As a result, (as an adult) I was blessed with the opportunity to create the EMBRACE program at Eskenazi Health in Indianapolis in June 2007. I couldn't bear knowing that there were women right here in our community that were facing cancer alone, and with very limited resources. I have been blessed to find many local organizations and individuals who have worked closely with us to support our patients throughout their journey as they fight this terrible disease. However, there has been one group that has not only offered love and support to our patients, but also hope and happiness in the midst of their pain.

We were so incredibly fortunate to have been introduced to Hello Gorgeous! of HOPE. There really are no words that can describe the happiness that our patients have experienced with this amazing group of extraordinary and talented people. A surprise day of pampering and a makeover is a thrill to any woman.

But, can you imagine the experience for a woman who is battling cancer and has NEVER had a makeover and has NEVER been pampered a day in her life!?!? Our patients struggle just to have access to food, medications and housing. A makeover would never even cross their mind as a possibility for them.

I recall one patient in particular who was chosen by Hello Gorgeous! of HOPE for a day of pampering. She was neglected and abused as a child and grew up in the foster-care system. She experienced homelessness as a teen and became a victim of domestic violence as an adult. She was on the verge of homelessness when we met her on the day of her diagnosis. She had stage 4 metastatic breast cancer. I can remember the terror in her eyes the moment she got the news.

We worked closely with this woman throughout her diagnosis and treatment. We were able to help her find a safe place to live, and were able to provide her with her medications and assist her with access to food and transportation; however, nothing that we did for her came close to what was done for her by the Hello Gorgeous! team! I will never forget the look on her face when she learned that she had been chosen for a day of pampering and a makeover. I don't think I ever saw this woman with such happiness in her eyes before or after that day.

It was so much more than just a makeover. It was a tangible representation of hope, love, faith, and value. It represented that she truly was a beautiful woman and worthy of something good. A woman with her history, even prior to cancer, seldom has the opportunity to experience emotions like this that deeply affect your self-worth, confidence, and feeling of being valued in this world.

I believe that her time with Hello Gorgeous! actually changed her life in her remaining days. When I saw her after that day, she walked a little taller and held her head a little higher. She smiled a little brighter and with more conviction. I genuinely believe that her spirit was changed because of the time, love, attention, and support she received from Hello Gorgeous! She became more at peace. It was almost as if she had waited all of her life for that one time when someone showed her that she really was a valued, beautiful, precious person.

THANK YOU, HELLO GORGEOUS! FOR GIVING HER THE GIFT OF A LIFETIME!

> DeAnna R. Wesley, MSW, LSW
> Director, EMBRACE Program
> Eskenazi Health, Indianapolis, IN

A Very Humble Thank You

Our family and friends are our most loyal volunteers and we can never thank them enough for all the help and support they show us every day. We would like to thank our parents, **Janice** and **Guy Chapman** and **John Becker**, for all that we have learned and the endless love and support they give to us every day.

To our **Creative Directors, Trisha** and **Dan Greenlee**, and their daughter, **Brianna**, for volunteering hundreds of hours each month to the cause and working with us every day to serve our women battling cancer, and the endless tasks it takes to do just that. You truly have hearts of gold.

To our siblings and their families, **Amy** and **Pat Hechlinski, Tina** and **Sean Frederick,** and **Maria** and **Jeremy Becker-Yates**; and to those of our family who have gone before us: **Jeanine Becker** (Mike's mother), **Larry Scanlan** (Kim's father) and **Sue Maggio**, for the love you always gave and for all you taught us along the way.

To our friends and mentors, **Tony** and **Tammy Magaldi**, for your unbelievable support and the foothold that you give us to continue with this project, when footholds seem very tenuous and sparse. You give us hope and build our faith. And you always greet us with a smile! Thank you for everything.

I again need to thank my sister, my assistant, my Affiliate Salon Coach and one of our Creative Directors of Hello Gorgeous!—all

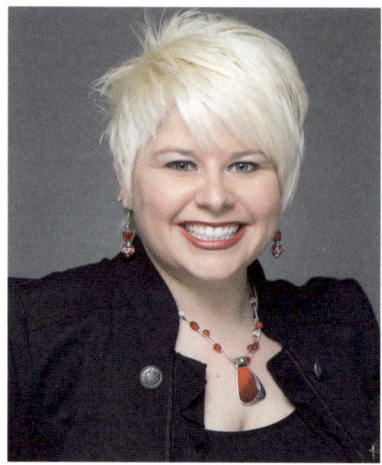

of whom happen to be the same person. **Trisha Greenlee** has been with Mike and me on this adventure since Hello Gorgeous! began. I would not want to do this without her and probably would not. Love you, Trisha.

To **Elissa Schmidt,** our **Art Director**, for her work on our book cover and all of the amazing and complicated projects that she uses her graphic talents so skillfully to complete. Thank you for always making Hello Gorgeous! shine.

To **Matt** and **Stephanie Slatner** at **PlanGenius**, for their wonderful work on our website and for their continued help in making it a hub of knowledge for all who visit our Internet site.

We need to thank the members of our talented Executive Team: **Trisha** and **Dan Greenlee, Julene** and **Javier Melendez,** and

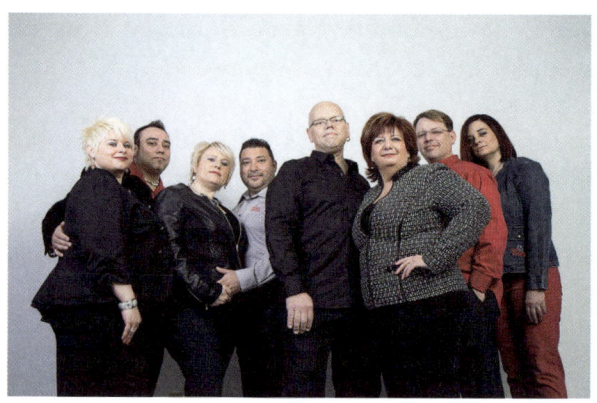

Thad and **Elissa Schmidt**. Their diverse and passionate talents, their gifts of ideas and counsel, and their sacrifice of time away from their families to participate in this project will always be one of our greatest resources. We love you all.

To **Diane** and **Larry Shoemaker**, for sharing your talents with us and for being wonderful mentors and helping us to develop every crazy idea we come up with.

To **Amy Reinert** and **Amy Reinert Photography** for your brilliant talent, your eye for detail and your giving heart in producing our cover photo and team photographs. Thank you, Amy. Your passion is showing!

To **Jeremy Stroup**, our videographer and film editor, for creating all of our How-To videos on the Internet. You have no idea how many people you are about to help with your talents.

Thank you also to our army of **Gorgeous Volunteers**. There are literally too many amazing people to mention, but especially people like **Julie Chrobot, Denise Longley and Darlene Tatay**, who help to further this cause in so many ways; whether they spend a single Saturday sweating with us as we work a Notre Dame concession stand or spend many months with the donations and details of a large fundraiser. These selfless individuals see the value of Hello Gorgeous! and always step out in faith to help.

To all our generous **Corporate Sponsors** who understand the need for our services and who donate their support for the sake and care of our Gorgeous Women. May your kindness and sacrifices return to you tenfold, blessing you in the years to come.

To **Jim Langford** and **Tim Carroll** from **Corby Publishing** of South Bend, Indiana, who made this book possible and have given us the opportunity to give this gift to all of you.

To **Josh** and **Isaiah** at **UR Phone Guy**, for your amazing work on the Hello Gorgeous! phone app, to help bring everyone to us with mobility.

To **Mark Borst** and **Chris Campbell** of **Cheveux Hair Salon** for their support and the use of their salon for video filming and Gorgeous Visits. Love you two!

A Special Thank You

This is a special thank you to some remarkable individuals and their companies that have stepped forward in faith to supply Hello Gorgeous! with the products and equipment to fulfill our mission for our women battling cancer. Their vision allows us to have purpose and impact and we are deeply indebted to them.

To **Dennis** and **Terri Falletti** of **Sella USA All-Natural Skincare** for their years of donating their world-class nanotechnology skincare to the hundreds and hundreds of Gorgeous Women who have gone through the Hello Gorgeous! experience.

To independent consultant **Kelly Taddeo** and director **Tricia DePauw** of **Mary Kay Cosmetics** for their singular efforts in raising tens of thousands of dollars in Mary Kay makeup, donated by hundreds of their customers, to be given to each of the women we serve through their visits in our Affiliate Salons throughout the United States. Do not ever tell me that two women cannot change the world, because I have seen it happen!

To **Dan Hnilicka** of **Graham Professional Beauty Products**, a division of **Little Rapids Corporation**, for approaching his company to donate all the key disposable spa components used during the Gorgeous visits to protect our women battling cancer from infection during their services.

To the **Paula Young Wig Company** for donating all the wigs and hats for every visit, and the promise through their foundation to continue doing so.

To **Matt Petrill, Mike Snell, Dave Watt and the owners, staff and craftsmen of Monaco Coach RV and ARG: Allied Recreational Group**, for their inconceivable generosity in the *complete* reconstruction of our 34' mobile DaySpa, HOPE, and for believable gift of our newest mobile DaySpa, the 36' 2012 Rambler Ambassador that they named FAITH. After 10 is, I am still speechless. You are all angels.

To **Jason, Melissa and the entire crew** from **Minerva Beauty Equipment** of Duluth, Georgia, for donating brand new spa equipment for our mobile DaySpas, to a non-profit, based 800 miles away from their location, sight unseen, as a result of a single phone call from Hello Gorgeous! When you look up "Faith" in the dictionary, it says "...see Minerva Beauty Equipment, Georgia."

There are so many other generous people who have stepped forward to help us through their products and services, too many to comprehend. People complain that there is less charity and caring in this world, but the best of humanity can be found by showing them the best of humanity in yourself. It has always surrounded this project, and words cannot express our gratitude.

"Be the change you wish to see in the world."
– Mahatma Gandhi

*"I believe in manicures.
I believe in overdressing.
I believe in primping at leisure
and wearing lipstick.
I believe in pink.
I believe that happy girls are the prettiest girls.
I believe that tomorrow is another day…
and I believe in miracles."*

– Audrey Hepburn

INTRODUCTION

If you are a woman, and you have ever heard the words, "You have cancer," *You Need This Book*. Within these pages are the conclusions to hundreds of questions asked by not only hundreds of the women battling cancer that we have served, but also hundreds of stylists and salon owners that have had clients sitting in their chairs, announcing quietly that they have cancer and that they need advice. These techniques are not taught in any beauty schools to this date: we saw a need for it and so we began asking questions and collecting information.

But, Why Should You Listen to Me?

If I were you I may be asking myself, "Who is this woman and why should I take any advice from her?" So I would like to share my experience with you.

Mike and I began Hello Gorgeous! in September 2005 as a calling, but, I have been a hairdresser for more than 25 years. I have been a national educator for a natural nail care company and an Italian color line; I have traveled throughout the United States and Canada, training other hairdressers on the techniques and benefits of each of these product lines. I have always felt that education in my field was very important, so I have traveled broadly to attend the best seminars and educational events in my industry, even attending the Vidal Sassoon Academy in London. I have had extensive training in haircutting, hair coloring, nail care, facials and seated massage in the hopes of becoming THE best hairdresser that I could be.

My husband and I then became salon owners, to pass this knowledge on to the next generation of hairdressers. Because dealing with the side effects of cancer on a beauty level is not taught in beauty school, we decided to talk with as many women going through cancer treatment as we could in order to find a way to combat their fears. We have done hundreds and hundreds of surprise makeovers on women with cancer, each of them with their own story and concerns. We have compiled the knowledge that we gained from each of those amazing women, and placed it in one complete guide for you.

We first saw the need for these services 17 years ago when my wonderful mother-in-law Jeanine was diagnosed with a glioblastoma in 1996. Michael and I knew nothing then and had very little help to offer her except for a few turbans and a lot of love. But, when we took up this calling in 2005, we began asking questions of the doctors, nurses and of the women battling cancer themselves. We began to ask about the physical symptoms of treatment; what the medical professionals saw and what the women experiencing cancer were feeling. Many of the effects of the cancer treatment that the women hated the most had to do with how it changed their appearance, not how they physically felt. And so we devised a program to help counter many of the cosmetic effects of the chemotherapy: hair loss, changes in complexion, dry, flaky skin, runny nose, loss of eyebrows and eyelashes. And we came to a conclusion.

Cancer steals everything feminine about a woman. It fills her with fear and threatens to steal her beauty, her joy and her life. This book is an easy-to-read, hands-on guide for all those women battling cancer to use cosmetic techniques that will help counter the side effects of chemotherapy and radiation on their beauty and their appearance.

The techniques of the Hello Gorgeous! Experience that we demonstrate in this book give you an arsenal of weapons with which to fight back. We have endeavored to explore every area of beauty that is important to a woman so that you, our Gorgeous Women, can step out into the public eye confident and empowered.

Because *every* woman deserves to be a Gorgeous Woman! When you see this note in RED:

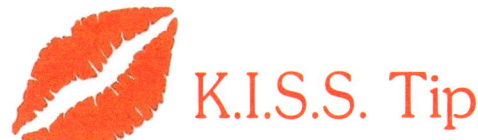 K.I.S.S. Tip

This designates a "Keep It Simple, Sister" Tip. These are simple, everyday beauty tips to keep all of us looking our best with skin care, nail care, makeup or just life. These are time-proven tips that will keep all of you the Gorgeous Women that you are. Enjoy!

DISCLAIMER

The information contained in this book should not be considered medical advice and is not a substitute for qualified medical advice. The information has been provided with the understanding that the author and publisher are not engaged in rendering medical, health, psychological, or any other kind of personal or professional services. The authors are trained cosmetologists, not medical professionals. The opinions expressed herein reflect the authors' personal experiences and ongoing investigations into ways to counteract the side effects of cancer treatments. At all times, the advice of trained medical professionals should be consulted before using any of the suggestions contained in this book.

 The information contained in this book is intended to provide helpful information for those dealing with the side effects of cancer treatment and their caregivers. The information contained herein, including all text, graphics, and images and all related materials are provided for informational purposes only. Although the authors make an effort to keep the provided information up-to-date, they cannot guarantee it.

The authors and the publisher specifically disclaim all responsibility for any liability, loss or risk, personal or otherwise, which is incurred as a consequence, directly or indirectly, of the use, application, or interpretation of any of the material contained herein. Reliance on any information provided by the authors is solely at your own risk.

THE GUIDE

Chapter 1

The Hello Gorgeous! Experience

Hello Gorgeous! is a 501(c)(3) not-for-profit that provides a red-carpet experience for all women battling all cancers, with full spa ambush-style makeovers in one of our 36' mobile DaySpas or by one of our partnering Affiliate Salons across the United States. Each venue delivers spa services and cosmetic education in a salon environment, at no cost to these Gorgeous Women. We have done hundreds of these makeovers, in a hundred different situations: from a visit in our first bus on a woman recently released from prison to a teacher nominated by her students, from an ex-Navy helicopter pilot to a grain-elevator secretary who twirled her skirt in front of a 10,000-person "Reveal." Each one is different, but ultimately the same, simple thing. It is about giving our attention to one woman at a time—one Gorgeous Woman at a time.

We began in our salon that we owned for 10 years. It all began with a calling.

> *"When the answer is simple, God is answering."*
> – Albert Einstein

Our Story

My name is Kim Becker and my husband Michael and I started this organization in 2005 as a calling. We owned a full-service hair salon in South Bend, Indiana, for 10 years. When we first thought to open the salon, my husband said to me: "I know what we should call the salon. We should call it 'Hello Gorgeous.'"

I promptly told him that was the stupidest thing I had ever heard in my entire life and that we were not calling it "Hello" anything! I had been an educator for a West Coast nail company many years before and had been very impressed by a salon there in which I had given several classes. It was a beautiful and elegant A-frame building—all glass—and they had served champagne and cheesecake to all their clients. It was called Cheveux, which meant "hair" in French, and I had known for the last four years that when I opened a salon I would call it that.

"No, no, it will be really cool," Mike said, "because every time you pick up the phone, if you greet the person on the other end with 'Hello Gorgeous,' it would make them feel good." I told him it was dumb and we weren't doing it, mostly because the name was already picked out!

We opened Cheveux Professional Hair Design and owned it for ten years. We grew the business quite a bit by the time we sold it. As in every business, we had our ups and downs between employees, taxes, wages, utilities and repairs. But I found that I just could not find the complete fulfillment in the salon that I very much needed.

There was just something missing. There was an emptiness that I could not explain. I thought that maybe there was something missing in me. So, I went to classes to further my education. I trained in Chicago and Miami and New York and I even attended Vidal Sassoon in London to train, which was one of my dreams. Still, I never seemed to find the fulfillment I was looking for. I became an educator for the color line that we used in our salon at the time, and I did a lot of traveling for them teaching classes. Many of the salons where I instructed on this particular color line were in downtown Chicago; top salons in the industry were asking for me as their instructor. Still I was not finding that fulfillment I was looking for.

I thought maybe a change would help. So we moved our salon across town, from one location to another, and tripled our size. We expanded our services and, over a few years, grew to 14 hair stations (with stylists and colorists from Beginner to Master), massage rooms, tanning beds, nail and pedicure rooms, esthetics room and multiple office staff. We did constant promotions, like referral programs, product sales for holidays, Back-to-School specials for product and services and "The Boss Is on Vacation" sales. We had *thousands* of clients and did a great business. Yes, it was coffee and mints, rather than champagne and cheesecake, but a wonderful salon regardless.

And still the emptiness was there. That is the only way I can describe it—just an emptiness.

In 2005, on a trip back from Indianapolis, Indiana, Mike and I were talking as our son Seth slept in the back seat of the car. I talked with Mike about that same thing that I had been feeling for a year or more—that I just felt like there was something else that we should be doing, that I thought there was a higher purpose for us. Suddenly I looked at him and I said, "I know what we're supposed to do!" Mike's eyes got big and he listened intently as he drove because he too was kind of down on our salon. It had been so much work all the time, for so many years, and it seemed like we just couldn't get it to where we thought it should be. He was looking for a higher purpose as well.

"We're supposed to have a mobile day spa, a mobile salon that will cater to cancer patients."

"Wow," Mike said, "that is unique. Wow."

"A place that will be a wonderful and peaceful sanctuary for them—a palace on wheels that will go to their curbside and pamper them with spa services and make them feel like a queen for a day."

"Yes," he said smiling, "that sounds amazing."

I told him we would offer these nurturing services to women with cancer: facial, manicure, pedicure, makeup and hair styling. I said that we could travel around Indiana doing these makeovers, making hundreds of women happy and changing their lives forever.

"YES!" he said again, louder. Mike was smiling more broadly with each idea, thinking of the positive impact we could make on all these people.

"And..."

"Yes?"

"AND..."

"YES?"

"And...and all the services we would provide these women would be free," I said. "We will charge them *NOTHING!*"

I watched all the color slowly leave his face.

"Kim, how are we going to *pay* for this? How can we make a living for our family?" he asked.

"I don't know. I don't know how it's going to happen, but I know it's what we're supposed to do." We spent the next few miles in the car with my trying to convince him that this is what we were supposed to do. Mike was not buying into it (I could tell) but, being the supportive husband that he is, he stopped at a bookstore in Kokomo and went inside the store to buy me three or four different books on "women and fund raising" and "women and nonprofits" and "grant writing for dummies"—anything he could find that would make this dream come true. He knew that, once I set my mind to an idea, there was little chance in changing it.

I spent the next hour talking about this and how we would make this happen. Mike was not saying much and he was changing the subject just about every chance he got. About 30 miles from home, our son woke up and we decided to take him into a play area so he could stretch his legs a little bit. As we were sitting there talking, I looked at Mike and I said, "You know what? *This* is supposed to be called 'Hello Gorgeous!' because, when these women feel the way that they do during their fight with cancer, that's how they deserve to be greeted. That's what they deserve to hear."

He still wouldn't talk to me about it and it took me several months to convince him. We held onto the salon for another year and then we sold it to concentrate our efforts fully on Hello Gorgeous. Since then, Mike has worked six days a week, 12 hours a day at this—for the last eight years. I work three days a week as an independent stylist, in the salon we sold to pursue this dream, supporting our family, as God unfolds this enormous and amazing journey in front of us. Every woman we are able to help teaches us something. The hugs and tears of joy tell us we are on the right path, that we are making a difference. And Mike has told me that, because of what he has seen with this project and what he has learned from these Gorgeous Women, even if he never gets paid real money to do this job, he will not quit.

I Promise to Put My Lipstick on…

So I wanted to share with you how this seed was planted for this book. I was at the salon getting ready to leave for a speaking engagement 30 minutes away. As usual I finished a little late so I was rushing around to tidy things up before I left. Now my sister Trish and I work together and she is a "Star." She looks perfect all the time. Her hair is done, and her makeup is on and she is always wearing red lipstick. And she is *always* reminding me to put on my lipstick. Sometimes it is just a quiet reminder, like handing me the lipstick. So that day as I was running out the door I said to Trish: "I Promise to Put My Lipstick on When I Get There!" Trish's eyes lit up like a Christmas tree and she yelled: "That is the name of your next book!"

   She was right!! We have taken more than 2 years to compile all of this information for you in order to give you the most complete guide to keep you looking Gorgeous! through your cancer journey.

So, Where Is "There"?

I stopped at a McDonald's at lunchtime one day to grab a quick salad, and I ate it in the parking lot. As I sat facing the local Harley Davidson store, I witnessed something that made me smile. I saw a woman in her mid-60s come out of the store and walk over to a beautiful red Harley. She straddled the bike like a pro, put her helmet on; then she took a tube of lipstick out of her hip-slung purse and put her lipstick on. Then she started that beautiful red Harley with a kick and rode away. I loved it—first things first. Always put your lipstick on, *even on your Harley.*

When we came up with the title of the book, *I Promise to Put My Lipstick on When I Get There*, we meant it to be an association—"there" is wherever you need to go at any particular moment in life, dependent on your situation. For a student, *there* may be graduation, or a new school, or grad school. For an expectant mother, *there* could be the birth of her child, or the first look of unconditional love. For a woman battling cancer, many times, the *there* that she is looking for may not be remission, as much as just a modicum of normalcy.

That is what Hello Gorgeous! strives to give—a handhold on normalcy. We give to you a way to feel that your world is not collapsing in around you—a *there* to head toward. We felt the need to write this book—to make sure that any woman going through this life-changing experience will never be alone when it comes to looking gorgeous throughout her cancer journey.

This guide will answer your beauty questions while helping you to feel "girlie" again, and helping you to counteract many of the side-effects that run hand-in-hand with your treatment program.

Over the course of my 25-year career as a hairdresser, I have been faced many times with a client sitting in my chair telling me that she has cancer. And, sometimes I was the first to know this information, even before anyone else in her family. She looks to me for guidance and advice on how to maintain normalcy in her appearance. I found myself reading what I could on the subject of beauty and cancer, which I found to be very little. So I went right to the source and talked to the women who have experienced cancer firsthand—finding out their fears, finding ways to calm them, and helping them to continue to feel and look like a woman (even when cancer can steal everything that makes you feel feminine).

When I was 23 years old, I had been a hairdresser for 5 years. I remember one of my long-standing clients coming in and telling me that she had been diagnosed with breast cancer. I was taken aback when she asked my advice as to what to do with her hair. I was not sure what to tell her. We were never taught this in beauty school and I do not remember ever seeing any classes on the subject. And *of course* she *would* come to me and ask my advice! I was her beauty consultant and, among other things, this process was going to change her looks drastically. I suggested that she purchase a wig, just in case, and told her that I read somewhere that, if she placed a bag of ice on her head during her chemotherapy infusions, her hair would not fall out. *What a wellspring of information I was!* Well, the ice trick did not work, so I am glad that she purchased the wig. When I think back to that day, I wish I had known then what I know now.

But I know it now and I am here to help. On the following pages I hope you will find all the answers you are seeking on beauty and cosmetics, whether it is for you or your loved one; and my sincerest wish is for you to come out healthy on the other side of cancer with a new outlook on life and that this book will change the lives of women with cancer in every nation—a new normal that will last you the rest of your long, full life. God Bless.

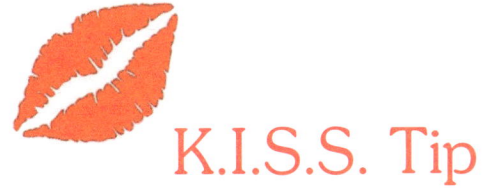

K.I.S.S. Tip

Talking on a cell phone can cause rashes along your cheek and jaw. Antibacterial wipes will keep your phone clean and help your skin stay clear.

> *"For I know the plans I have for you,"* declares the LORD, *"plans to prosper you and not to harm you, plans to give you hope and a future."*
>
> – Jeremiah 29:11

Chapter 2
Attitude First

Before we begin with the physical parts, let's touch on the mental game. The old saying that beauty is only skin deep is a misnomer. As my husband Mike would say, Beauty at a distance can be just a pretty face, but Beauty close up has a lot to do with character and attitude. Illness, and the survival through it, also has a lot to do with attitude. I have known people who frown and carry on like a child for days about a stubbed toe. And I have known women battling cancer, nauseous from chemotherapy, who could light up a room with their smile. Attitude is a choice, and it is an advantage more for you than for the people around you. It can get you through situations that no drug or supporter can.

"Just because I laugh a lot...doesn't mean my life is easy.
"Just because I have a smile on my face every day,
doesn't mean that something is not bothering me.
"I just choose to move on and not dwell on all
the negatives in my life.
"Every new moment gives me a chance to renew anew.
"I choose to be that."

– Anonymous

What You Focus on, You Become

Let's start with focus. I am embarrassed to say that I used to think this was malarkey. I was convinced that I could easily think and say negative things and still be a positive person and still achieve a positive result. Then I started to pay attention.

Really pay attention.

Have you ever noticed that the car that you have dreamt of owning is now everywhere that you look? What about the new Coach bag you would love to have? Now it seems like everyone has one. You don't believe me? Okay, take three minutes to do this exercise.

Set your watch alarm or kitchen timer for three minutes, press go, and then look around the room that you are sitting in, look for everything in the room that is blue. Blue. Blue, blue, blue. That is what you are looking for: Blue—every shade of blue—dark blue, light blue, azure, cobalt, teal, sapphire, robin's egg, royal blue. Blue. Okay, got it? After you read this next sentence close your eyes and think of everything you saw that was...

GREEN!

Did you feel it? Could you think of something that was green? Blue was your focus so my guess would be you could not. This is so true with our lives. When you focus on one thing, you are blinded to another; focus on the negative and that is all you see. Try this for a day—look for the positive in everything that you see. Do not speak one word that is not positive—no gossip, no criticism, no self-reproach.

I know that this can be hard, especially when you are going through cancer treatment. There will be times that no matter how hard you look, there seems no positive side to a certain situation. But I can tell you that there always is.

My husband Michael is a wonderful man and my best friend. We have been married for 20 years and we have a 12-year-old son. Three years after we were married, Mike was diagnosed with a very rare liver disease. This man has had countless procedures, hundreds of IVs and 18 years of hospital stays, too many to even count. In the last six years, Mike has been in the hospital every six months for an elongated stay. I have never seen a fighter like this man, but not once has he asked, "Why me?" Each stay he tells me, "It will be okay. There must be a reason that I need to be here."

As strange as this might sound, Mike often tells me that he is grateful for his disease. He says that he is thankful for where he is, for what he has gone through, and that he would not trade his disease for anything. He has learned too much about life, and about himself through the journey—his *there*, if you will.

Through our journey with Hello Gorgeous! we have met so many amazing and inspirational women. Mike always looks at me with a big smile and says, "I'm the luckiest guy walking!" Mike easily could have given up years ago or he could have become very cynical and bitter, as so many people do. But instead, he spends his time making a difference in other people's lives. To look at him, you would never know anything is wrong; because, to Mike, dealing with his disease is just business as usual.

You can either be bitter or better. It is your choice and it is up to you.

> **"Skilled sailors aren't made on smooth seas. If you aren't headed into a storm, currently in the middle of a storm or just coming out of a storm, you are doing it wrong. Only dead fish go with the flow."**
> – Dana McDonald, RD, CNSC, LD
> Eat Clean, Train Mean, Live Green

Attitude Is Everything

Janis is a very sweet woman that we met at an ovarian cancer event in Indianapolis. She is a middle-school teacher who loves her career and her students. By the time I met Janis, her cancer had returned for a second time. She has an amazing spirit and a wonderful attitude. She thinks of her cancer as a chronic disease that needs to be treated on a regular basis, much like diabetes. In her mind, it is not a death sentence. It is just an inconvenience. I *love* that thought process. Her cancer does not keep her from living.

Lynne was another gallant woman that I had the honor of serving. She made a deal with God that she would take all the cancer that He needed to give her, in order to keep her three sisters free of it. Lynne was diagnosed with cancer three separate times. She claimed that each reoccurrence was protection for one of her sisters. Each time, she took the diagnosis in stride and held her head high. She never lost her grace, her poise or even her smile. Cancer could not take any of that from her.

In battles like these amazing women are waging, attitude really is everything.

Ultra Efforts

Now I am not much of a runner. I actually think that people who run for fun are a little crazy. I have attempted training to run a 5k and that is still on my bucket list. I would like to know that feeling of accomplishment—the feeling you have when you cross that finish line and you know that all of your hard work has paid off.

And there are so many different runs. There are 5k, 10k, half-marathons, full marathons, and there is an ultra-marathon. Now the half-marathon is 13.1 miles, the full marathon is 26.2 miles, and an ultra-marathon is 26.2 miles or more. I love what my husband says: "I only run when chased." I have talked with many of these runners, people who have run multiple marathons, and I asked them, "What gets you through? How do you keep going when you feel like you cannot run another step?" They tell me it is all a mental game. You just keep telling yourself that you can do it and you push yourself harder and longer than you ever have before.

My friend Holly ran 50 miles in one day. No, that is *not* a typo. Fifty miles! She did this to raise funds for Hello Gorgeous! (in honor of her friend Kathy, who received a makeover in October of 2012, but then lost her battle with ovarian cancer in February of 2013). Kathy had an amazing spirit of determination. We were lucky enough to be there for Holly's first step of the 50 miles and we were there for the last step, as she finished her 50 miles. At the end of 36 miles she looked great, like she had just gone for a casual stroll. But the last 12 miles for her were grueling. She told me that her mind was great, but that her body was giving out.

As I watched her stretch and rest periodically along the route, all the while pushing herself beyond anything I could imagine, I wondered what was going through her mind. What did she have to tell herself to keep going? There was no prize money for her at the finish line. She was giving all of the money she had raised away. It was just amazing to me. Not once did she consider giving up. Not once did she think of taking a short cut. No one would have known but her.

Holly was in this for the long haul. She needed to say that she did it. She won this contest against herself.

I started to think that cancer treatment is much the same thing. I imagine that cancer is much like an ultra-marathon. Not just your normal jog or even a pleasantly run 5k, it is the longest run you will ever take. And there are some of you who have had to run this ultra-marathon more than once. It is a mental game. Your body may start to fail, but you have to talk yourself into finishing. Just when you think you cannot take one more round of steroids, one more needle stick, one more radiation treatment; you have to tell yourself that you can! You have to finish. You need to beat this and say that you have won!

Holly's Story

When my dear friend Kathy Gribbin was diagnosed with stage 3 ovarian cancer, my mind seemed to go numb. A small group of her friends and family gathered in the waiting room while she was in surgery. Her oncologist came out to tell us the news, and I recall thinking how strange it was that while she slept, we were finding out her tumors were malignant. I tried to imagine how she would respond to the diagnosis and I realized that, despite our friendship of 16 years, I couldn't predict how she would face this.

For the next three years, Kathy taught me what it truly meant to live an optimistic life. I gained so much perspective as she continued to mentor college students, travel, plant flowers, and fill her social calendar. Kathy wore bright colors to her chemotherapy treatments,

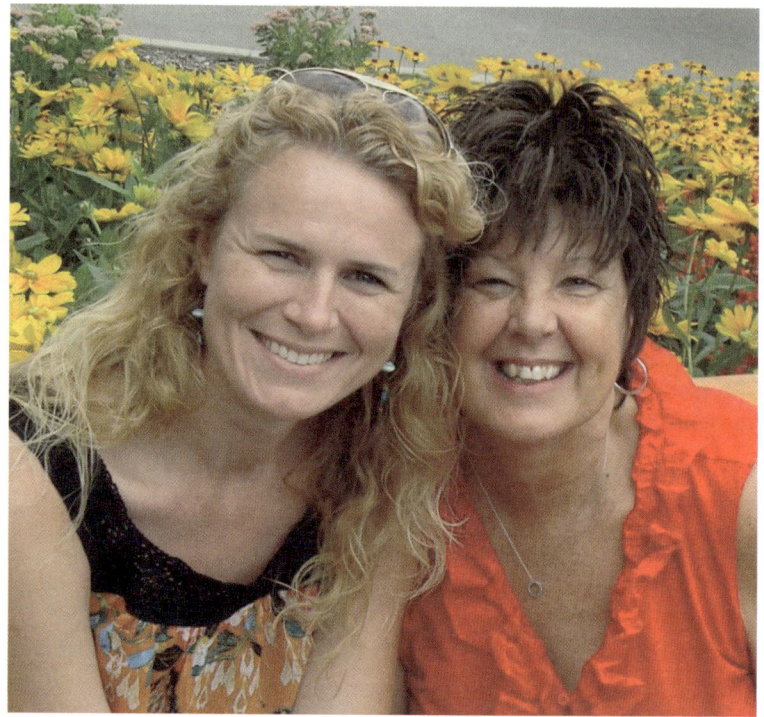

Holly and Kathy

and toted chocolate chip cookies with her to give to the nurses. In her blog she once wrote, "I am not sure all that God wants to teach me on this journey—but I will do all I can to have an open heart and mind!"

I looked for ways I could make life better for Kathy. Then one day, an incredible opportunity presented itself to me. I was invited to a Hello Gorgeous! open house at a salon called The Beehive. I met Kim Becker and her sister, Trisha Greenlee, as I toured one of their mobile day spas. Trisha explained their mission to pamper women fighting cancer, and my eyes welled up as I told her about Kathy. I was sure she would love to be a makeover recipient! So Trisha gave me her business card and explained how to nominate her. A few weeks later, I got the call that Kathy was chosen. We surprised her at work and swept her away to The Beehive for a full morning of spa treatments. There was so much anticipation in the weeks leading up to her makeover—and the actual event itself was even better than I imagined! Kathy's feistiness and humor made it a fun morning for everyone, and by the time her makeover was complete, her true, bright self had emerged.

That was the last day many of her friends saw her look so vibrant. Her health quickly declined. And three months later, she passed away. It was so difficult to comprehend how someone who lived with such true purpose and meaning could be gone. One of Kathy's missions on earth seemed to be to encourage others to pursue their dreams. So I decided I would pursue one of my dreams in honor of Kathy.

I loved what Hello Gorgeous! did for her—and for her loved ones. Following Kathy's makeover, she and I had talked about how I could get involved with Hello Gorgeous! and my mind kept going back to my love for running. I had run 15 marathons, but I dreamed of one day running a 50-mile ultra-marathon. My uncertainty—whether I could run that far—made me want to try. A month after Kathy died, I said it out loud: "I'm running 50 miles to raise money for Hello Gorgeous!" That made it a reality. I called it "The Live-Fully 50," in honor of Kathy. I talked about her a lot as I explained why I was training, and this helped me work through my grief in a way I didn't expect. It was so positive and productive. I know Kathy would have liked that.

There were days, though, when my nerves would get the best of me, and I'd worry that 50 miles was too lofty a goal. More people than I expected were jumping on board and donating—the money steadily poured in. It was so exciting, but nerve-wracking, too. In the midst of training, I was babying a strained hamstring. What if I couldn't finish and had to return everyone's donations? I couldn't mentally camp out there for too long. I prayed, got massages, prayed some more and trained some more. I figured out that I had to take the training one day at a time, thinking only of the task in front of me that day, then writing the miles down in my training calendar with satisfaction. I needed to be my own best cheerleader if I wanted to succeed. People would say, "I don't even like to *drive* 50 miles!" Well, honestly, neither did I! But Kathy deserved a tribute that was big. And so did Hello Gorgeous!

The day of the run was finally here, and I was ready to stop thinking about it and just *run*. I had been feeling so nervous as the day approached, but surprisingly I woke up with a sense of calm that I immediately acknowledged as the "peace that passes all understanding." God was answering the prayers of my loved ones.

I had planned four 12.5-mile loops around town, beginning and ending each one at The Beehive. A very enthusiastic group of friends and family was at the starting line; even a local news station covered it. I couldn't believe all the hoopla surrounding this event—but I welcomed it! The energy worked wonders on me.

I ran the first and second loops with focus, but with a light heart. It was a great day. I didn't wear a watch because I wanted to cover the distance in my own time; no pressure. During the third loop, my legs ached but I still felt strong. My friends went out of their way to muster up support all over town, even from strangers! On a street where people were dining alfresco, one by one they stood up and clapped for me as I ran by. Then, on the campus of Notre Dame, students lined my route and cheered. Someone even played the Notre Dame fight song on a trumpet! My heart was bursting. I didn't have room in my head for any negative thoughts! Thank God for the enthusiasm of others. It is so powerful.

As I approached the end of the third loop, I was relieved to get a break and to stretch. I ate, visited with friends, got a good, quick rubdown, and made my way outside to run. When I was taking those steps toward the door, I knew this final loop was going to be harder than the previous three loops combined. Despite the stretching, my muscles felt intensely tight. Stiff. Then, as I slowly began to run, I imagined how awkward my form must have looked. It was time to dig deep. I had to put those 37½ miles I had just run out of my mind. It was time to concentrate only on the actual stretch of road I could see in front of me—not the turnaround point ahead, not even the finish line—only that short distance directly within my scope of vision. My mind was still strong. I just felt like I was bargaining with my legs: *Just to the next pole; now, to that corner—soon, you won't have to do this again for a long time.*

Is this how Kathy felt when her body wouldn't cooperate? This seems like such a false comparison to me now, but on that road,

I think it was the closest I had ever come to understanding her fight. Her positivity seemed to empower her to get through each treatment, one by one. Despite her fatigue, she somehow would engage her chemotherapy nurses in conversation. When I went with her once, I could see that they were in awe of her bright spirit. She lived in the moment. And those moments added up to three challenging but very good years. I needed to live in the moment too. On that last loop, Kathy felt so near to me as the sun went down. I trudged forward believing she was smiling on me from a place where darkness never falls.

A massage therapist who treated me for the first time just two days prior to the run somehow sensed my pain. He and his wife are on the Hello Gorgeous! Executive Team. They found out where I was on the course and ignored all speed limits to reach me! Julene opened the trunk of their van, folded down the seats, and I lay down. Javier massaged my weary legs. I set out to run again; then a few miles later, I had to walk. Javier gave me another massage. Because of him, I could run the remaining distance. They then led the caravan of vehicles driving slowly alongside me. Their headlights illuminated the way. What a comfort!

Then about two miles from the finish line, two fire trucks pulled up beside me. A friend who is a firefighter arranged for them to escort me through downtown to the finish. Because of those men, I didn't have to stop at a single red light! I knew I had to ignore the pain and just keep moving. Supporters were waiting in the rain for me half a mile from the finish and, when I passed them, they ran behind me, cheering me on. What love! I have never felt as loved as I did on that day. It's what helped me push away the pain and finally cross that finish line. I was so happy! I had accomplished my goal. That truly was the best day of my life.

People continued donating even after I finished. I am still slack-jawed when I think of the generosity that was poured out. The gifts to Hello Gorgeous! on behalf of my run totaled $17,049.24. Wow! So many makeovers!

I will never stop missing Kathy. I wish she could have been physically present when I ran those 50 miles. But my heart is full because she inspired me.

A Positive Attitude Is Contagious!

Joyce Meyer, the evangelist, has a good saying. It is a constant reminder to me on a regular basis.

"You can be bitter or better."

It all depends on you. You are the master of your own attitude. It may be the one thing over which you have control. So how will you use it? In many of the good women that I've met along this journey, their cancer diagnosis has come out of the clear blue sky. And it hit them like a proverbial ton of bricks. Many of these women have shared with me that on the day of their diagnosis, they were first in shock and then they were in denial. They told me that they just could not believe this was happening to them. Many women told me that they asked, "Why me?"

Then something rises up inside of these women. It is a fighting spirit that they did not know that they had in them. They put on their boxing gloves and do something that they had never had to do before. They fight the fight of their lives, for their life.

Everyone fights differently. Some fight quietly and in solitude. They do not let anyone outside of their immediate circle know what is happening to them. And then, there are some who rally every person they know into their corner. Their belief is that there is strength in numbers. The amazing thing is that there is no right or wrong way to fight. It is all about what works for you. You just have to fight.

Cancer is a beast—mean and nasty, indiscriminate and heartless—but you can fight and you can win.

I can say that I do not have this experience firsthand. But I have talked with hundreds of women diagnosed with cancer. Each one takes up a different weapon and fights in her own way. It is your choice to be bitter or better. I love the weapons that one of our Gorgeous Women, Kristie, uses to fight. She is officially known as "Wonder Woman" in her circle of influence.

Kristie was treated with chemotherapy and radiation. Her chemotherapy lasted 16 rounds. Kristie looked at this as 16 opportunities to celebrate! She gave each session a different theme. There was "Mardi Gras," "St. Patrick's Day," and a "Pink" theme, complete with feather boas and big pink floppy hats. I attended

Kristie's last chemotherapy, which was a "Hawaiian" theme. It was a huge party that day. Of course, Kristie had enough props to share for every person. What was not inherently fun, Kristie and her spirit made into a fun occasion.

On one of her treatment weeks, Kristie took the money from a fundraiser that she had held and paid the medical co-pays of everyone coming to clinic that day. Her joy and spirit rubbed off on everyone in the infusion center on her party days. So what will you choose? How will your story read?

Will your attitude be better or bitter?

How Can a Positive Attitude Affect Your Health?

According to the *Huffington Post*, studies have shown that an attitude—positive or negative—can affect our health. A positive attitude can also provide benefits to our health and well-being.

Some of the ways are:
- Reduced risk of death from cardiovascular disease
- Greater resistance to the common cold
- Greater mental and physical health and well-being
- Increased life expectancy (par. 3)

No one can *make* you mad; you *choose* to be mad—so choose *not* to be mad. Smile because laughter is the best medicine and humor improves immune cell function.

You have to take the initiative to inject humor into your life. Some suggestions are:
- Read a blog post that makes you laugh
- Hang out with friends who never fail to boost your mood
- Start a conversation with "What was the funniest thing that you ever did?" Or "What was the funniest movie you ever watched?"
- Go to the park with your dog
- Play dress-up with your kids

Anything that is going to bring a smile to your face is good medicine.

Positive Affirmations

What are positive affirmations? These are positive phrases which you repeat to yourself. These words describe how you want to be. Positive self-talk is crucial for success, especially the success of beating this disease. You have to "think positive." Think good healthy thoughts; imagine yourself whole and enjoying a long, healthy life.

Each year we take a retreat at the beginning of the year with our Executive Team. We make plans on how to grow our organization to be able to help more women. We also try to help each of our team members to grow as individuals. This year we created an exercise that would pump each member up daily.

We gave them a stack of 2"x3" text cards that were connected at one corner by a ring. We asked them to write a positive affirmation on 25 of the cards. Each of the affirmations needed to begin with "I AM." We then asked them to place them on their nightstands and to read these each and every morning as they woke up before ever getting out of bed. We knew that this would start their day on a positive note.

These ideas are based on sound, solid medical facts and deal with the science of neural biology. The joining or wiring together of brain cells is often referred to as "cells that fire together, wire together"; and the theory explains that, when we learn, groups of cells that are activated together grow a stronger connection. This group of common brain cell gives us learned behavior—walking, talking, running, singing, etc.

What Are You Smiling About?

I love to smile. I love making other people smile. And, as I have come to find out, smiling is good for you. According to About.com/Healthy Aging, here are the top ten reasons that you should smile:

1) Smiling makes us attractive.
> We are driven to people who smile. There is an attraction factor. We want to know a smiling person and figure out what is good in them.

2) *Smiling changes our mood.*
   The next time that you are feeling down, try putting on a smile. There is a good chance that your mood will change for the better.
3) *Smiling is contagious.*
   When someone is smiling, they lighten up the room, change the mood of others, and make things happen.
4) *Smiling releases stress.*
   Stress can really show up in our faces. Smiling helps prevent us from looking tired, rundown, and overwhelmed.
5) *Smiling boosts your immune system.*
   Smiling helps the immune system work better. When you smile, immune function improves possibly because you are more relaxed.
6) *Smiling lowers your blood pressure.*
   When you smile there is a measurable reduction in your blood pressure.
7) *Smiling releases endorphins, natural painkillers, and serotonin.*
   Together these can make you feel good. Smiling is a natural drug.
8) *Smiling lifts your face and makes you look younger.*
   The muscles that we use to smile lift your face and make a person appear younger.
9) *Smiling makes you seem successful.*
   Smiling people appear more confident, are more likely to be promoted, and are more likely to be approached.
10) *Smiling helps you stay positive.*

  Try this test. Smile. Now, think of something negative without losing the smile. It is hard to do when we smile because, although our mind is attempting to hold onto a negative thought, our smile is sending out the message to the rest of our body that "life is good." (par.1-3)

It takes fewer muscles to smile versus frowning and it takes more effort to frown than it does to smile. So try it...SMILE!!!

What a Smile Can Do!

As I mentioned earlier, my husband has been in and out of the hospital for a long time. For many of these hospital stays, we were at Indiana University Medical Center in Indianapolis. On one particular visit, I tried an experiment.

Now my favorite pastime is to "people watch." You can learn so much just from watching other people. Once Mike went into his procedures, I was by myself for the duration. I would take a walk, usually to the cafeteria. On my way to the cafeteria I noticed that no one looked happy. Quite frankly, they all looked miserable: doctors, nurses and visitors. Now I know that the hospital isn't my favorite place to be either, but I can usually find a ray of sunshine in every situation. I bought my beverage and returned to the waiting room to wait for the word that Mike's procedure was finished. Two hours later he was in recovery and I decided to return to the cafeteria. But this time I decided to smile at everyone I saw along the way, just to see what happened. I was amazed at the reaction. Nine out of ten people smiled back. I hope I was able to spread a little joy that day.

So keep smiling. As they say, it makes people wonder what you have been up to, and it can obviously change their mood, as well as yours.

Laughter Is the Best Medicine

According to HelpGuide.org, there are health benefits of humor and laughter. Humor is infectious and laughter is contagious. Laughter also triggers healthy physical changes in the body. Humor and laughter strengthen your immune system, boost energy, diminish pain, and protect you from the damaging effects of stress. Best of all, this priceless medicine is fun, free, and easy to use.

Laughter is a powerful remedy for stress, conflict, and pain. Nothing works faster to bring your mind and body back into balance than a good laugh. Humor can lighten your burdens, inspire your hopes, and keep you grounded, focused, and alert.

Laughter relaxes your whole body
> A good hearty laugh releases physical tension and stress, leaving your muscles relaxed 45 minutes later.

Laughter boosts your immune system
> It decreases stress hormones and increases immune cells (infection-fighting antibodies), which improves resistance to disease.

Laughter triggers and releases endorphins
> The body's natural feel-good chemicals, endorphins, promote an overall sense of well-being and can even relieve pain temporarily.

Laughter protects the heart
> It improves the function of blood vessels and increases blood flow which can protect you against a heart attack. (Par. 1-3)

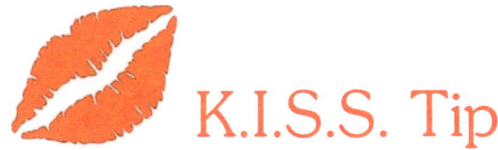

K.I.S.S. Tip

Smile with your eyes. A wholehearted smile will naturally draw in the eyes. This natural smile is called a Duchenne smile. It's not something you can fake; when you're forced to smile for photos, your eyes don't smile. It's only when you truly feel like smiling that you flash a Duchenne. The eyes are essential for a genuine, warm smile.

> ***"Your sense of humor is one of the most powerful tools you have to make certain that your daily mood and emotional state support good health."***
>
> – Paul E. McGhee, Ph.D.

Chapter 3

Comfortable in Your Own Skin

Let's begin with skincare. Your skin is the largest organ of the body and, dependent upon the area of skin, it can absorb from 60 to 100 percent of what we use on it. This section will guide you and give you the information you need to have beautiful, radiant skin during your cancer journey.

It will give you hints and tips on how to keep your products uncontaminated when your immune system is compromised. It also covers the power of touch and ways to help nurture your skin, to establish an effective skincare routine.

> *"Beauty, to me, is about being comfortable in your own skin."*
>
> – Gwyneth Paltrow

History

According to Lexli.com, "the [practice] of self grooming…[has its] origins since ancient times. People have…endeavored to make themselves more attractive… [M]en and women have used an endless variety of materials and substances as cosmetics for the skin and hair.… (par. 1)

"During the reign of Elizabeth I (1558-1603), facial masks were in vogue. Formulas for lotions and [masks] were made from such ingredients as powdered eggshell, alum, borax and ground almond and poppy seeds. Milk, butter, wine, fruits, and vegetables were also used in cosmetics…" (par. 5)

J.K. Knowles writes, "The ancient Egyptians were avid bathers and experimented with many formulas for skincare products. For example, a natural exfoliator was a mixture of sand and aloe. This applied not only to people of status, but to the common people as well. All Egyptians were expected to maintain a standard of hygiene, and workers were often paid in body oils that were used by both women and men to protect their skin from the hot sun and dry air." (par. 1, 2)

Many women we have met have not experienced facials on a regular basis. They have told us they feel that this service is for the rich and famous. And many tell us that they do not deserve this level of pampering. I strongly disagree. Everyone deserves to be and should be pampered, even if it is only every once in a while. Facials also serve a purpose during your cancer treatment. They keep your skin moist and vibrant and can help replace nutrients and repair the damage your skin may encounter during treatment.

Dry Skin

My friend Barb found regular facials very beneficial to her. Barb and I have been friends for a very long time. We attended grade school and high school together.

In February of 1998 Barb was diagnosed with a stage 3 Anaplastic Astrosytoma—a brain tumor in the right front lobe of her brain. They gave my friend 18 months to live. They treated her with the strongest dose of medical radiation that a human can receive and then four rounds of chemotherapy. The radiation was so strong that the hair on Barb's head from her ears forward never grew back. And it left a very nasty radiation burn on her forehead that the dermatologist said would never go away. Believe it or not, that is what Barb was most self-conscious about. The radiation burn left her forehead red, very itchy and dry. It flaked constantly.

I suggested to Barb that she start coming in once a week for facials. We decided that she had nothing to lose. We performed weekly facials for a five-month period, then bi-weekly facials for two months, then down to one time per month. And, it worked! The radiation burns disappeared. Her skin was silky and it glowed. When Barb returned to her dermatologist, the doctor could not believe what she saw. Barb has told us how much more confident she now feels, even though her hair has never regrown. Her forehead still looks great! And she has been cancer free for 16 years!

Skin care is very important during your cancer treatment. A good skincare system can be your best friend. Unlike your makeup regimen, where you can use one brand of foundation and another brand of blush, it is very important to use all of the same products for your skincare regime. The system will work together for good and keep your skin looking as healthy as possible during a very taxing time. Chemotherapy often causes dry, irritated skin.

WebMD.com offers these tips to prevent dry skin during treatment:

- Skip long, hot showers.

Hot water strips oils from the skin faster than warm water. Long showers or baths can dry out your skin. Limit yourself to a single five- or ten-minute warm shower or bath a day.

- Use a gentle cleanser or shower gel with moisturizer.

Instead of harsh cleansers, go for unscented, soap-free, or mild soap cleansers.

- Moisturize while skin is still moist.

Pat your skin with a towel after you shower or wash your face or hands, leaving the skin damp. Apply a moisturizer within three to five minutes of washing to lock moisture in. (par. 2)

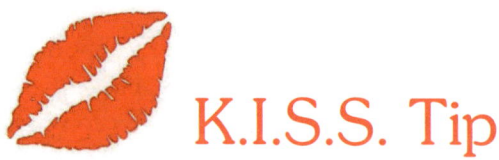 # K.I.S.S. Tip

A consistent, smart moisturizing routine helps. Wash with a non-soap liquid cleanser, preferably one with ceramides to replenish the skin's outer layer; pat skin dry for less than 20 seconds and apply a thick moisturizer to slightly damp skin within minutes of bathing to trap in moisture.

Why Is Skincare So Important?

Your skin is your body's largest organ. It serves as a protective barrier between your insides and the rest of the world. It also helps regulate body temperature.

Your skin is in a constant state of growth: old cells dying and new cells forming. Healthy skin appears vibrant and full. Avoid using hot water when you wash your face as the heat sucks the moisture from your skin. Try warm or cold water instead.

According to Jennifer Freestone, a Yahoo-Network contributor, whatever you put on your skin is absorbed in 26 seconds. The skin has a pH of 5.5, which is mildly acidic. If your skincare products are not pH balanced they can strip away the protective layering that is there to balance your skin. (par. 4)

Cleansing

Cleanse the skin to remove dirt, makeup and pollution. This should be the start to every skincare regimen and should be done twice daily—once in the morning and once at night. If your skin is dry, you can skip the morning wash and use a soft cloth and water to refresh your face in the morning. Always use a gentle touch and circular upward movement.

Danielle Page at TheExaminer.com shares with us:

Top 5 reasons not to wear your makeup to bed:
1. It creates a breeding ground for bacteria.
2. It clogs your pores.
3. Leaving grime or sweat or dirt on your face overnight will cause further free radical damage to your skin, which wouldn't occur had you taken it off before bed.
4. Because the skin repairs itself at night, it will not have the essential vitamins and moisturizers to enhance the repairs that it would have had if you had cleaned your face before going to bed.
5. Leaving mascara on your lashes overnight will dry out your lashes and make them brittle. If this is done too many times, they may fall out.

Toning

My feelings are that you need to be careful with toning. Chemotherapy, radiation and steroids can make your skin dry and irritated. Many toners and astringents have a good amount of alcohol in them which can leach the moisture from the skin and leave a burning or strong tingling sensation. There are some toners that have very little alcohol in them and can be "misted" on to the skin with a spray bottle.

Look at the ingredients on the product label. The closer the word "alcohol" is to the first few ingredients, the more alcohol there is in that product.

Moisturizing

1. Moisturized and healthy skin slows down the signs of aging
2. It keeps your skin healthy and soft
3. It will keep your skin as moist as possible during your chemotherapy and radiation treatment. (par. 1-3)

Tom Scheve on Health.HowStuffWorks.com explains that "Moisturizers come in two forms: humectants and emollients. Humectants draw water into the outer layer of skin (the epidermis), from the middle layer (the dermis), as well as from the environment. Glycerin is an example of a humectant. Emollients are moisturizers that leave the skin feeling smooth and soft while sealing existing moisture to the face. Emollients can be oil-based or water-based... Most moisturizers are emollient creams that contain humectants, so you won't have to choose between the two." (par. 2)

Applying a moisturizer prevents water that is already present on the skin from evaporating. For this reason it is important to apply moisturizer within about three minutes of bathing. Lightly pat your face dry after washing, and then apply your moisturizer.

Putting a moisturizer on a dry face will prevent external moisture from reaching the skin and keeps the skin drier.

Applying Your Moisturizer

When I apply my moisturizer I use the "Dot Method." I place a dot on my forehead, on each cheek, one on my nose and one on my chin. Using a circular motion and an upward movement, I massage the moisturizer into my face. I feel that I can more evenly distribute my moisturizer this way. When applying eye cream under your eyes, always use your ring finger. It is the weakest of your fingers. Use a light touch and a patting motion, moving toward your nose. Because you are not stretching sensitive skin around your eyes, this movement will save you on crow's feet.

Hydrating Your Skin Is Paramount!

In 2011, I had the opportunity to meet a wonderful woman by the name of Morag Currin. Morag is the president of Touch for Cancer and the founder of Oncology Esthetics. She authored the books, *Oncology Esthetics: A Practitioner's Guide and Health-Challenged-Skin: The Esthetician's Desk Reference.*

Oncology Esthetics has become the leading oncology skincare training in the world. This training integrates the knowledge of traditional cancer treatments and the possible side effects, together with the necessary skills and modifications to ensure that safe spa treatments are performed. I find her to be extremely knowledgeable when it comes to the subject of challenged skin, especially while going through cancer treatment. Morag states that, "For many people undergoing cancer treatment skin issues occur, many times with frustrating outcomes. The focus of the patient and the medical team is essentially, that of patient 'survival,' so skin issues do not appear to fit into a priority sequence." She goes on to say that "From a skin care professional's perspective, and the psychosocial aspect of a person, skin is the most visible organ to others and any imperfections create additional stress to the cancer patient. Keeping an array of skincare products to the bare minimum is necessary during treatment, as the body is already overburdened with medications. The focus needs to be keeping the skin barrier as intact as possible so hydrating, protective skin products are necessary."

Treatments for Your Skin

There are treatments that can aid your skin in a more youthful appearance. These procedures can be performed by an esthetician or a doctor. The following procedures should be performed on a healthy person, but I would suggest *not* during active cancer treatment.

Microdermabrasion is a non-chemical non-invasive procedure that uses a spray of micro-crystals to remove the outermost layer of the dry, dead skin cells and reveal a younger, healthier-looking skin layer. Microdermabrasion also encourages the production of a new underlying layer of skin cells with higher levels of collagen and elastin, which improves the skin's appearance. Microdermabrasion is much gentler than dermabrasion.

Dermabrasion is a more intense procedure used to treat deeper facial lines, extreme sun damage, and scars.

Chemical peel is a body treatment technique used to improve and smooth the texture of facial skin using a chemical solution that causes the dead skin to slough off and eventually peel off. The regenerated skin is usually smoother and less wrinkled than the old skin. Chemical peels are sometimes used to treat certain types of skin cancer.

Again, unless a chemical peel or microdermabrasion protocol would be prescribed by your oncologist (which is very rare), I would suggest avoiding these services while undergoing your cancer treatment.

Don't Touch

Celebrity Esthetician Renée Rouleau states: "Touching your face all day long, without intentionally doing so, is making your face one of the dirtiest parts on your body. It's important to clean the skin to avoid the spread of acne bacteria that can cause increased blemishes."

Wash your hands before you wash your face. Do not use the family hand towel that has been hanging over the rack for several days. Bacteria can breed on the towel and be transferred to your face and neck. Gently pat your face dry with a disposable towel that is soft.

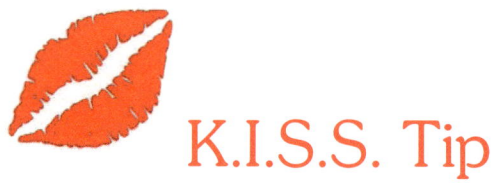 K.I.S.S. Tip

The best time to apply lotion is right after a shower or bath, when skin is still damp. Moisturize your hands every time you wash them so that evaporating water doesn't draw even more moisture from your dry skin.

"I love to put on lotion. Sometimes I'll watch TV and go into a lotion trance for an hour."

– Angelina Jolie

Chapter 4

Can't Touch This... or Can You?

Massage is a service that we originally had in our program but use very little due to the ports, scarring and the surgeries that patients experience during their cancer journey.

But touch, and the power it has to comfort, console, and heal a person is very real and sorely needed, especially during an illness. Here are some of the advantages to touch and the balm that it can be to a cancer patient.

"Nothing is so healing as the human touch."
– Bobby Fischer

Touch

Massage can be a very "touchy" subject. (Catch the pun?☺) When we first started performing our surprise Hello Gorgeous! Makeovers, we had included chair massage into the program. I love massages, I love giving massages and I love receiving massages. One of the businesses that we owned was called Relief In-Site. We were an on-site massage business that performed stress relief chair massage for major corporations. It was very fulfilling to work on someone for 15 to 20 minutes and have them stand up and look refreshed and renewed.

I have had extensive training in manual lymphatic drainage, massage for TMJ and for carpel tunnel syndrome. I felt very comfortable performing seated massages. But when it came to massage and women with cancer, I felt that I was under-trained, so we removed it from our program.

When it comes to massage, I would recommend talking with your oncologist. Ask their opinion and get a referral to someone that is certified in oncology massage. There is a right way to do things and a wrong way to do things. Massage therapists who are trained in oncology massage know how to comfort you, treat your tight areas, relieve your stress and tension, and still keep you safe and on your treatment plan to perfect health. Oncology massage is safe and effective at helping people feel better during challenging times. Find a qualified massage therapist, and you'll be on your way to a peaceful reprieve from the stress of cancer.

Oncology Massage

According to Tracy Walton, a specialist in massage therapy, massage is safe for people living with cancer, "when practiced by a skilled therapist with background or training in massage and cancer." (par. 1) When using massage therapy on people battling cancer, therapists need to know: how to work with complex medical conditions; how to conduct detailed interviewing; joint movement; and, when to consult with the client's physician for needed information.

You want to look for someone who has one of the following in their résumé:
- Advanced training in oncology massage
- Specializing in oncology massage
- Massage for people with cancer
- Massage therapy for oncology support (page 4, par. 5)

Benefits of Human Touch

All talk of professional massage aside, touch is a very important part of your cancer journey. According to Carmen Jochmann in "Benefits of Human Touch" at Suite 101.com: "Touch is the first sense to develop in the womb and the last sense to leave in old age. It is essential to the health and well being of human's emotional, physical and mental development. It is so vital, in fact, that therapist and author Virginia Satir stated that human beings need:

four hugs a day for survival,
eight hugs a day for maintenance and
12 hugs a day for growth." (par. 1) *(italics added)*

How many hugs do you receive each day? How many hugs do you give each day? I am a "huggy" person. I attribute that to my upbringing. For the 25+ years that I have been a hairdresser, there are very few times that a client has left my presence without a hug...whether they wanted one or not. It was as much for me as it was for them.

The benefit to a person's health is phenomenal. Touch can reassure you, relax you and comfort you. Touch reduces depression, anxiety, stress, physical pain and it can be very healing. Touch also increases the number of immune cells in the body and has powerful effects on behavior and moods.

Touch is vital to the positive health and development of all human beings regardless of age. Humans need to touch and be touched just like they need food and water. It is a way of communicating, lifting spirits and experiencing happiness in our lives. Without it people will experience sadness, loneliness and isolation.

According to Cari Corbett-Owen at Ditch-Diets-Live-Light.com: "Research done in both the 19th and 20th centuries shows that *when babies aren't touched they literally waste away and have problems with the development of their bones....*" (par. 7)

"Research done with adults shows that *regular touch lengthens our lives and cuts down on doctors' visits. It releases serotonin and oxytocins and reduces cortisone—touch is a great stress reducer.*" (par. 8)

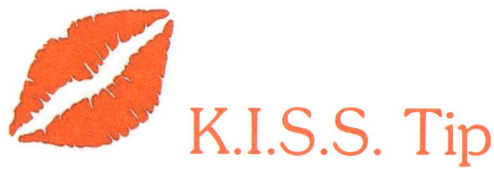

K.I.S.S. Tip

When you are touched by another person, the signals sent to your brain translate into feelings of security, *happiness*, and comfort. These feelings are supported by a *decrease in stress* hormones and an increase in oxytocin, a hormone thought to calm and counter stress.

> ***"A hug is a universal medicine, it is how we handshake from the heart."***
> – Anonymous

Chapter 5

Nails...
Your Second Best Feature

This section covers everything about nails, manicures and pedicures. And there IS a story behind the title. The nail industry is growing—in 2000, there were 50,000 nail salons in the US, compared to over 200,000 nail salons today. And it is an easy and impactful way for you to feel good about yourself, and change your appearance.

"It's all fun and games until someone breaks a nail!"

– Anonymous

History

According to the internet site WiseGeek.com, "The history of nail painting dates back to the Chinese, when as early as 3000 B.C. royals used a variety of substances including flower petals, beeswax, egg whites, silver and gold to tint their nails. In Egypt, both men and women colored their nails, with color indicating social status. The royals used darker colors for painting their nails, while the lower classes used paler tones." (par. 5)

They also discuss the fact that nail painting in America first became a fashion statement in the 1920s—with the introduction of paint for cars. Before that, women would tint their nails with red oil or they added gloss with tinted creams or powders. The painting of women's nails was popular in France before it became popular in the United States. By 1925 women who wanted to paint their nails could do so with a rosy red color, which was generally applied to the center of the nail but not the moons.

Actress Rita Hayworth made the look of long red nails very popular in the 1940s. It was not until then that the average American woman dared to paint her nails. Look how far we have come!

Fat Women Look Better with Long Fingernails

I once met a woman who was a bit overweight. She told me that she had tried every diet and spent hundreds of dollars trying every diet pill on the market to lose the weight. Every attempt was unsuccessful. So, one day she made the decision to quit dieting and concentrate on growing her nails long because she said, "Fat women look better with long nails." This made me smile and I thought about it for myself. I do feel better when my nails are manicured and polished. It makes me feel *finished*.

Why Is It Important?

Many years ago I had heard that it was proven that the first thing the majority of people look at when they meet someone for the first time is their eyes. And the second are their hands. The condition in which you keep your hands and nails, your jewelry, whether your hands are smooth or careworn, tan or pale, whether you have your nails manicured or you are a nail biter—all of these signs can make a statement about your social station, the type of job you hold, whether you are a person who settles or you are an achiever. As they say, details create the big picture. And the condition of your hands and nails can send a loud message.

But paying attention to these details can have a positive effect on you as well. Again, do not ask me why, but I do feel better when my nails are manicured and polished. It makes me feel finished and pampered. And taking the time to do these things for myself makes me feel like I matter.

Do these sound like thoughts and attitudes that come up during your battle with cancer?

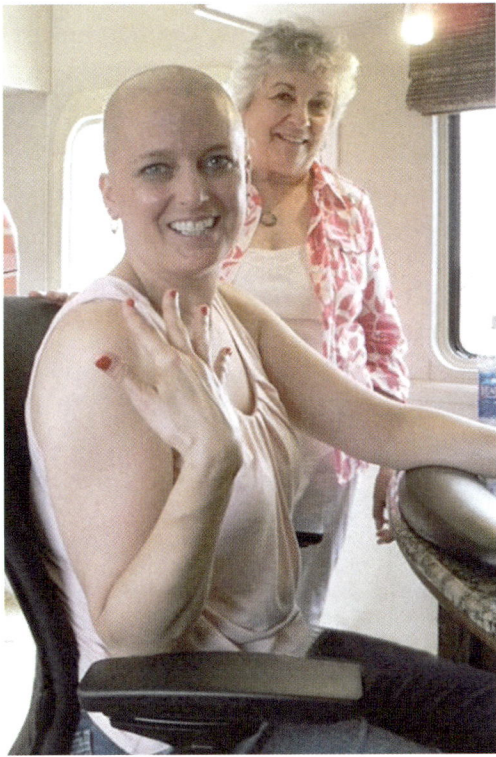

Elise feeling "finished"!

Aunt Sue's Story

When we first started Hello Gorgeous! we wanted to be able to tell the story of what we do—what comprised Hello Gorgeous! What was it all about?

My Aunt Sue was going through breast cancer at that time and we were helping her through her battle by fitting her with wigs; supporting her through her appointments and her chemotherapy treatments; and giving her advice on makeup, skincare, and other concerns. It was around then that we had the idea of having a pictorial visit to show what Hello Gorgeous! did for these special women and so I asked Aunt Sue if we could use her to tell our story.

She would come to the salon and we would pretend to give her a Hello Gorgeous! visit. We would take pictures of each step to create a storyboard. And that is what we did. When we began that day, because of the time constraints of filming, we manicured one of her hands, took the pictures throughout the service, then

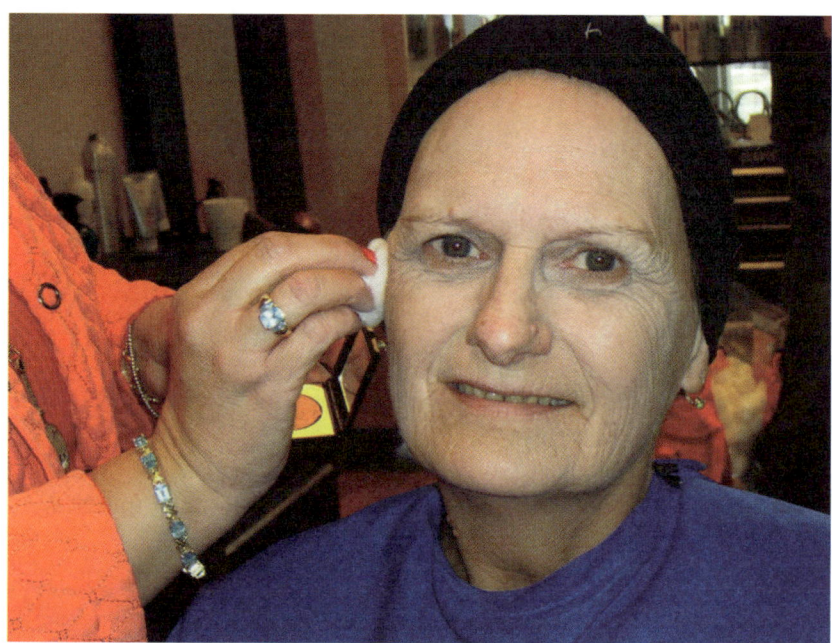

just painted the nails on her other hand to match and moved on. We did the same with the pedicure—performing the full service on one foot, taking pictures, and then painting the other toes to match. For the facial we put her mask on, took the pictures and took the mask off. We applied her makeup and I had her bring a different outfit from home to change into, then we took the "after" pictures. It was fun and we created some awesome memories from that day. But what I did not know was how much that abbreviated visit meant to her.

The next day was Easter Sunday. I will never forget it. My Aunt Sue came up to me and gave me a huge hug. She told me that she lay in bed that morning for an *extra* 30 minutes just remembering how special we had made her feel the day before. I was so surprised! My response was, "Are you kidding me? We used you!" She hugged me again and thanked me over and over.

Six months later she revealed to me that she was still wearing the chipped and tattered remnants of the nail polish that we had put on her toenails that special day before Easter. Every time that she looked down at her toes, as chipped as the polish was, she was reminded of that day and how special she had felt. It was then that we knew we were on to something.

From the Nail Files...

It is a known fact that the first thing a person looks at are your eyes and the second thing they look at are your hands, whether it is looking to see if you are a nail biter or if they are looking for a ring to see if you are "taken."

Chemotherapy has a job, a big job, and that is to kill all of the fast growing cells in your body, because that is what cancer is—a fast growing cell. However, it also kills many other fast growing cells, including those that make up your nails.

Through your cancer treatment, your nails may become hard and brittle. They may discolor or even start to lift.

Here are a few things that you can do to ease the trauma that may occur to your nails:

Use cuticle oil

Massage cuticle oil onto the cuticle of each nail. The oil will absorb into the tissue and this will help to keep the cuticles from becoming dry and splitting. Apply the cuticle oil at night right before bed. The molecular structure of the oil is more readily absorbed at night. This will give you the most benefit. While applying the oil, massage each nail with a circular motion for a count of 10 for each nail. This will also encourage growth.

Use lotion often
This will help to keep your skin soft and help keep it from cracking. Keep lotion in your purse, your car, your kitchen and your bedroom.

Keep nails short
If the nail becomes thick and hard, keep the nail trimmed short. This will help avoid hitting the nail, which may crack or tear the nail.

If the nail begins to lift
Gently file the nail to blend the thick nail in with the new nail. Keep fingernail polish on the nail even if it is just "clear." This will help seal the lifting and help avoid a fungus from growing in the nail.

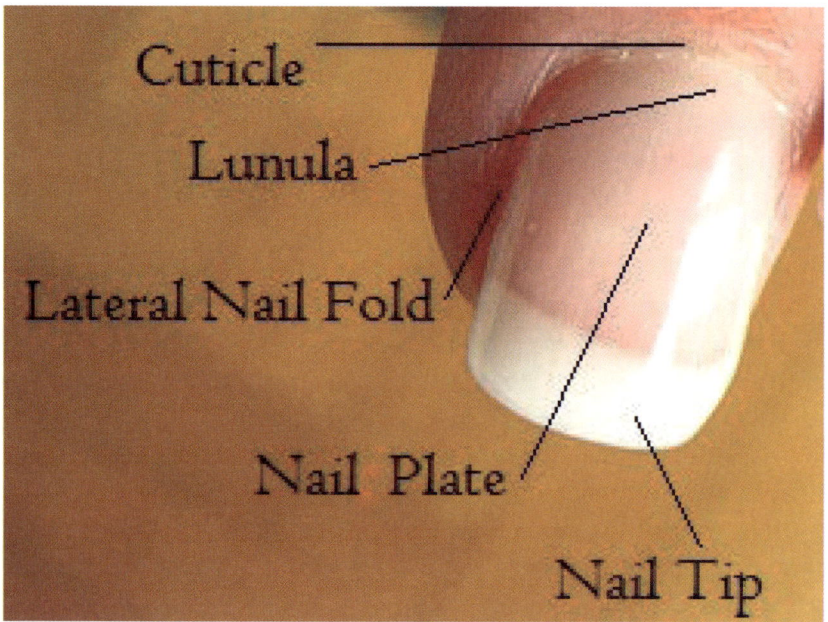

The Correct Way to Remove Length from Your Nails

If your nails start to show damage from your cancer treatment, such as peeling, splitting down the center of the nail, or if they become brittle, the best thing to do is to keep them short until the damaged portion of the nail has grown out. Your nails will be easier to maintain and will prevent further damage if you keep them at a shorter, more manageable length.

There are two ways that length can be removed from your nails:

1. An emery board or fingernail file can safely remove length from your nails. When filing your nails, you want to remember to move the file in only one direction. You never want to "saw" your nails or move back and forth. This will cause friction, which can cause more ripping or tearing of the nail.

    Always soak your nails in water first, or trim your nails after a bath or shower. This makes the nail more flexible and easier to trim.

2. When trimming the nail down, you can use nail clippers and, yes, there is a correct way to do this as well. When trimming your fingernails, you never want to start trimming at the center of the nail. You want to start with one side of the nail, then clip the opposite side of the nail, leaving a point, then clip the center of the nail, removing the point. If you clip the center of the nail first, you can cause a tear at the side of the nail close to the skin. This area of the nail is the weakest area. Trimming the nail in three parts will help to preserve the strength of the nail.

    The nail may be extremely brittle due to your cancer treatment. It would be extremely difficult to trim this type of nail with one snip. Cutting the nail in three clips will make it easier to clip the brittle nail without causing any further damage to the nail.

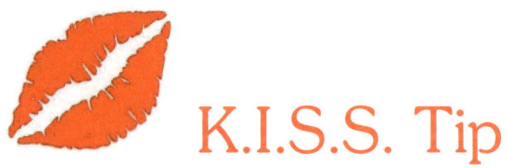

K.I.S.S. Tip

Try to use fingernail polish remover only once per week. Polish remover has alcohol in it which can be drying to a normal nail. We need to protect your delicate nail. Rather than remove the polish as soon as it chips, reapply color polish and a top coat over the existing polish until it is time for the weekly removal. Try using non-acetone polish remover—it is less drying to the nail.

Always Use a Base Coat

A base coat will protect the nail and prevent the color polish from staining it. A base coat will also set a better foundation and help the color last longer. Apply one coat of the base coat, two coats of color and one coat of top coat to seal it. And, if your nails are brittle, avoid nail strengtheners at this time.

Does Nail Polish Really Help My Nails?

Nail polish protects the nails from becoming dry, flaky or breaking. Nail polish creates a barrier or a shield over the top of the nail, giving the nails a smooth, hard coating that protects the nail from splitting and allows the nail to grow.

Gently Push Your Cuticles Back

The best time to push your cuticles back is right after a shower or bath. The cuticles are soft and pliable and are less likely to rip or tear when they are wet. Wrap the end of your towel around your thumb and use it gently to push back the cuticle on each of your fingers. Switch thumbs and perform the action on each finger of the other hand.

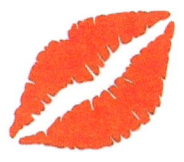 # K.I.S.S. Tip

Fingernails are known to grow 1/10th of an inch per month. If you lose a fingernail it could take 4 to 6 months to regrow completely. But your fingernails do grow 3 to 4 times faster than your toenails.

Acetone versus Non-acetone Remover

I love wearing nail polish. I feel more finished when my nails are painted. I usually change my polish once a week. If done correctly, that should be often enough for anyone. You can keep your manicured nails looking fresh by applying an additional coat of top coat every other day for 7-10 days. Then remove the polish and start fresh. So, that being said, what is the best way to remove your polish? Below are the differences between acetone and non-acetone polish remover. While going through cancer treatment, I would recommend non-acetone polish remover, as it is gentler to the skin and nails.

Acetone Polish Remover

Acetone is a powerful solvent that removes nail polish quickly. It is a clear, harsh-smelling solvent that is highly flammable. This solvent is strong enough to disintegrate some plastic.
- Acetone polish remover is a powerful solvent that removes nail polish easily;
- Acetone polish remover can be very drying to the cuticles;
- Acetone polish remover should not be used on acrylic nails;
- Acetone polish remover can be drying to the nails as well;
- Acetone polish remover should be avoided if the nails are dry and splitting.

Non-acetone Polish Remover

Non-acetone polish remover contains no acetone. It does, however, contain ethyl alcohol, a less aggressive solvent. This is not as strong as acetone polish remover, so it may take longer to remove your polish.

- Non-acetone polish remover is gentler on the skin;
- Non-acetone polish remover can be used on acrylic nails;
- Most non-acetone polish removers will add moisturizing agents like glycerin to minimize the drying effect of the polish remover on your cuticles and nails;
- Non-acetone polish remover requires more effort to remove polish, especially dark colors;
- Non-acetone polish remover is best for frequent polish removal, light colors and women with dry or more sensitive skin and nails.

Acrylic Nails

My personal opinion is to stay away from acrylic nails. You need to protect yourself. I feel that between filing, buffing and the chance of fungus setting in due to lifting, I would suggest avoiding acrylic nails during treatment.

Now there are exceptions. If you have a nail technician that you trust, and they can take their time with you and be extremely cautious, and if you take your own buffer, file and orangewood stick, I would say okay. However, you really need to watch the lifting on your natural nail. This can cause the acrylic nail to lift, which can be an opening for fungus or bacteria.

What to Do if Fungus Starts

Consult your physician. There are many oral and topical medications that will help get rid of the fungus or the bacteria.

How to Find the Best Nail Shapes

You may not even know that there are different ways to shape your nails. There is no right or wrong shape. It is whatever fits into your comfort zone. Did you know that you can use the shape of the half-moon at the base of your nail to determine the best shape for the free edge of your nail?

According to Allwomenstalk.com, there are five basic nail shapes:

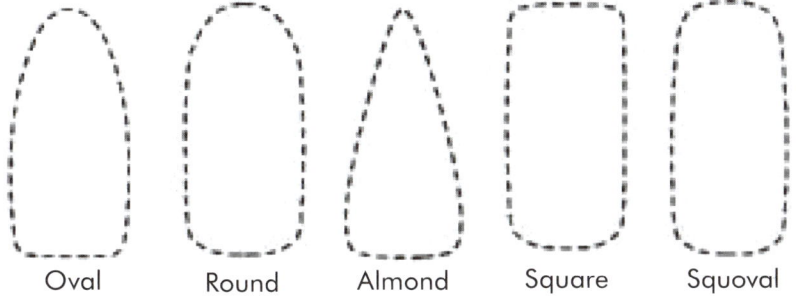

Oval   Round   Almond   Square   Squoval

Oval
This shape looks good on most nails. Oval gives you a classic base to polish on your favorite shade. This nail shape is durable and it looks great on both medium and long nails.

Round
With a round nail, your hand will look proportioned and poised. This is an ideal shape for someone who has weak nails and likes to keep them short.

Almond
This shape will elongate your hands and give you a classy look. This is the weakest natural nail shape. This shape is very feminine and gives the hand a more delicate look, but this shape does not allow the nail to grow much.

Square
This shape balances out long fingers and draws attention to your hands. The shape looks best on medium or long nails.

Squoval
This look goes perfect with everything. It is the best of both worlds; a square nail with rounded edges. This is the perfect combination of square and oval.

Manicure? Why, Yes!

A short nail that has been manicured looks much better than a short nail that has not been manicured. I hear so often, "My nails are too short to get a manicure." I disagree with that statement. A short nail that is shaped, cuticles that are pushed back, and nails that are polished look beautiful—long or short.

While in treatment, how can I protect myself while getting a manicure?

1. If possible, visit a Hello Gorgeous! Affiliate Salon in your area for your manicure. The stylists at a Hello Gorgeous! Affiliate Salon have been trained on how to keep you safe and give you a memorable experience.

2. If you are unable to find a Hello Gorgeous! Affiliate Salon, I would recommend going to a well-established professional hair salon that offers manicures and take your own personal manicuring items with you:
    + orangewood stick
    + a nail file
    + fingernail polish remover pads
    + base coat
    + top coat
    + favorite nail color

    a. Wash your hands before the manicure begins. This will remove any unwanted bacteria in the instance of a nick or cut during the service.

    b. I would ask the manicurist *not* to use nippers on your cuticles during the manicure. Even the smallest nick or cut can become a breeding ground for bacteria. No matter how skilled the manicurist is, accidents can happen. If the use of nippers is avoided, then we avoid an accident.

    c. If you do get a nick or cut during the manicuring

service, wash your hands immediately with antibacterial soap and water for at least two minutes. Then apply a small amount of triple antibiotic cream to the affected area.

K.I.S.S. Tip

For best manicure results, apply thin layers of product. Start with a thin layer of *base coat*, apply a thin layer of polish down the middle, then one on the left and one on the right. After the first coat dries for a few minutes, repeat, then follow with a thin layer of *top coat*.

Neat Feet – Pedicure

The same precautions that are taken for your fingernails should

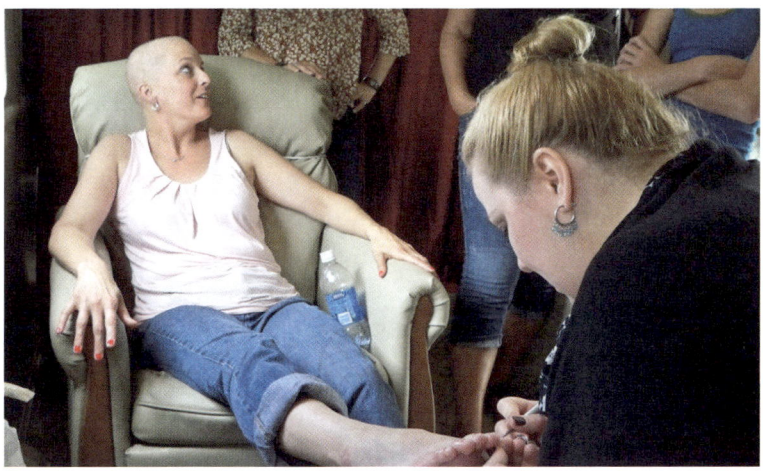

be used for your toenails. Keep your feet moisturized to prevent cracking and peeling of the skin on your feet.

Keep your toenails trimmed short. You may also lose your toenails during your cancer treatment. Your fingernails grow three to four times faster than your toenails, so it may take your toenails a bit longer to grow back.

If you visit a salon to have a professional pedicure, take these steps to protect yourself:

1. If possible, visit a Hello Gorgeous! Affiliate Salon for your pedicure. The stylists at a Hello Gorgeous! Affiliate Salon have been trained on how to keep you safe and give you a memorable experience.

2. If you are unable to find a Hello Gorgeous! Affiliate Salon, I would recommend going to a well-established professional hair salon that offers pedicures and take your own personal pedicure items with you:
    - orangewood stick
    - a nail file
    - fingernail polish remover pads
    - pumice stone
    - base coat
    - top coat
    - favorite nail color

    a. Soak your feet in a soapy scrub before your service. This will soften the cuticles and calluses, and remove any unwanted bacteria in the instance of a nick or cut during the service.

    b. I would ask the pedicurist *not* to use nippers on your cuticles during the service. Even the smallest nick or cut can become a breeding ground for bacteria. No matter how skilled the pedi-curist is, accidents can happen. If the use of nippers is avoided, then we avoid an accident.

    c. If you do get a nick or cut during the pedicuring service, wash your feet immediately with anti-bacterial soap and water for at least two minutes. Then apply a small amount of triple antibiotic cream to the affected area.

    d. Avoid the use of callus shaving tools at this time.

All these hints and tips should allow you to enjoy the health and pampering of a manicure and pedicure during the time of your cancer treatment. These are just simple precautions to keep you safe—and cut, nip and fungus free.

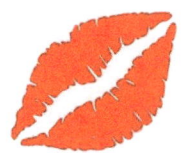

K.I.S.S. Tip

Your nails are jewels, not tools. Treat them kindly. Wear gloves when doing the dishes or yard work, and they will shine bright like a diamond!

> *"Beauty is how you feel on the inside and it reflects in your eyes."*
>
> – Sophia Loren

Chapter 6

The Balder the Head, the Bigger the Earrings

Okay. Here it is: the part of the cancer journey most despised by women—hair loss. Losing your hair can be one of the scariest symptoms during your journey, because it is a direct attack on one of the physical attributes that make us stand out as feminine.

But, in these next few chapters, we will help calm your fears about hair loss and hair substitution, and give you the tools to boost your image confidence. Remember, for most of you, this is a temporary condition. I cannot promise your hair will return exactly the way it used to be, but it will return. And we are here to help you with the transition!

"We're all born bald, baby."

– Telly Savalas

So Where Do the Earrings Come in?

The title of this section is "The balder the head, the bigger the earrings." Okay. My mom taught me from the time I had my ears pierced at a young age that you are not completely dressed until you have your earrings in. "It completes your look," she would say. I cannot tell you how many times I have left my house, after forgetting to put earrings in, and gone back home to get them before starting my day.

Now that you have had some hair loss, I would wear earrings every day, all of the time. It keeps the girl in you out in front and foremost in your mind. So go get yourself some fun, big earrings. If people are going to stare, give them something to stare at!

Why Is Hair So Important to Women?

The Examiner.com states that in a documentary film produced by Chris Rock, Maya Angelou states: "Hair is a woman's glory." Even as far back as Ancient Egypt, a woman's hairstyle indicated her age, status, role in society, and political importance.

Diva's, Inc. states that our "hair is an extension of who we are... Hair is intimately connected to our self-image, and when it looks good, it makes [us] feel good." It shapes our face and makes our features stand out. So, when there is a chance that it may be taken away, it can hit us hard emotionally.

2 Millimeters

So there may be some of you who are reading this book and the thought will cross your mind, "Why even bother?" or "I have no hair, no eyebrows and no eyelashes. How can any of this make the least bit of difference? HOW???"

I am going to share with you a story from someone whom I consider to be a mentor, Anthony Robbins—a wonderful motivational speaker. Tony talks about "the 2 Millimeter Difference"—how two millimeters, even though a very small thing, can make all the difference in a situation.

Tony told a story about a plastic surgeon friend of his that was considered the top in his field, and was flown all over the world to work on some of the most famous faces out there. As Tony sat waiting for the doctor in his office, he noticed a book of pictures. These pictures were of beautiful men and women. He noticed that adjacent to the different parts of their faces the doctor had placed numbers, as if they were measurements. Tony came to find out that this doctor had mathematically figured out what made gorgeous people gorgeous and other people, well, not so gorgeous.

For example the doctor had calculated that on a drop-dead gorgeous woman, the distance between the top of her upper lip and tip of her nose was the same distance as the width of her eye. Only a one-millimeter difference, either way, and the look of the woman becomes average. A two-millimeter difference and the woman is considered unattractive. Now, I have not tried this to see where I fall. I am not sure I want to know. But my point is that one millimeter can make a very drastic difference—two millimeters, an even bigger difference. I know you have days when you don't feel well—you might even feel downright lousy—but put on a little lipstick, put in some big earrings and brush a little blush on your cheeks.

Two millimeters *can* make all of the difference, trust me!

Just to give you the concept, there are approximately 25 millimeters in one inch!

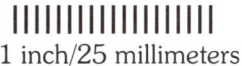
1 inch/25 millimeters

Lori's Story

When Lori was diagnosed with breast cancer, a big concern for her was the loss of her hair. Lori is a high school teacher at a prominent military academy. She wanted to make a seamless transition into a wig to make sure that the students in her classes were comfortable with her appearance.

Lori's doctors told her that she had a 50/50 chance of losing her hair. She wanted to be proactive, so we found a wig that was close to her current style and we sent the wig home with her before she began her treatment, just in case the chemo started to win and her hair began to fall out. Two weeks after chemo began, Lori started to lose her hair. She called me and told me that she was ready.

She came to the salon with her daughter and we shaved her head. She felt empowered from the precautions we had taken and decided to have a little fun. I shaved the breast cancer ribbon into what was left of the hair on her head. She wore it with pride, but her wig was ready whenever she felt the need.

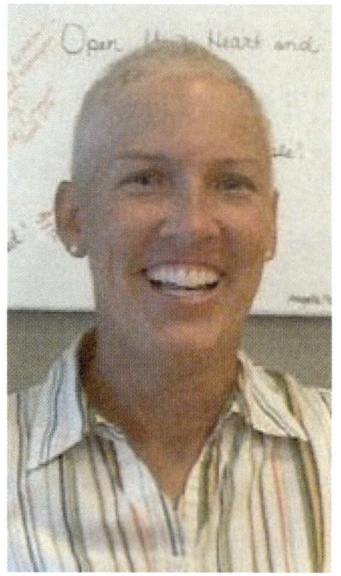 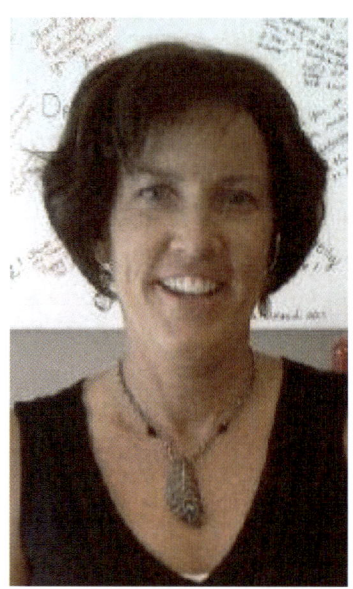

Lori Before   Lori After

Personal Preference

When my aunt was diagnosed with breast cancer, we cut her hair into a shorter style so that it would be a bit easier for her when her hair started to fall out. But as cumbersome as it was when her hair was falling out continually—having to pick up her own hair from all over her house and her clothes—she never wanted to shave her head. She wanted to keep as much of her old self as she could. And that is okay.

Consequently, when my friend Lori was diagnosed with caner, her approach was different. As soon as her hair started to fall out, she wanted to shave her head. She wanted no part of watching it fall. She wanted to be in charge and take care of it herself, before the chemo did. That is okay, too.

I have discovered that there is no right or wrong way to do this. It is completely *a personal preference*. I would like to educate you on what we have found to be helpful in this area.

Not all chemo will make you lose your hair. Chemotherapy is designed to kill fast-growing cancer cells. It also ends up killing many other fast-growing cells that make up your hair, eyelashes, eyebrows and fingernails. In order to kill the bad, some of the good has to be killed as well. I have found that breast cancer patients who take chemotherapy as part of their treatment almost always lose their hair. In other cases, the hair can be affected but not necessarily lost. If the hair stays during treatment it may become dry or brittle, even change colors to a lighter or darker color. Here are some steps you can take to make this transition easier:

1. Decide if you want a wig.
2. If you know that hair loss is a possibility, it may be easier to cut your hair into a shorter style. If the strands are shorter, it can be less traumatic when the hair loss begins.

Give people something to look at other than your bald head or changing hair. Find some really big, fun earrings. Wear a different pair every day—something that makes you feel sassy and girlie. Remember, the balder the head, the bigger the earrings.

Shaving Your Head

In my many years of doing Hello Gorgeous! and my experiences of helping hundreds of women who are battling cancer transition their looks, I have shaved a lot of heads. And I can assure you that, when you make the decision that it is time to shave your head, there is no right or wrong way to do it.

- You can make an appointment at a *Hello Gorgeous! Affiliate Salon* and have it shaved by one of our Makeover Specialists.
- You can go to your salon and have a professional stylist shave it for you.

- You can have a head-shaving party and allow your children, friends, and family to shave it for you.
- Or, as one of our fantastic Gorgeous! Women did, you can turn on some comforting music, pour yourself a glass of wine, borrow some clippers and have your own, private moment.

One of our Gorgeous Women, Anne, wanted me to shave her head as both her daughters were sitting in the next chairs in the salon getting their updos for Prom! There really is no wrong or right way to do this. This is your head and your fight, and you can do it however you see fit. If you choose to shave your head, the amount of hair you leave there is also your choice. When I shave a woman's head, I start with the longest setting on the clippers that I can use and still remove hair. I then work my way shorter, changing the guards. That way, she can tell me when she is comfortable with the length, or when to continue.

The whole purpose of shaving your head is so that you are not shedding all over your house, your car, and yourself; and that you are not constantly bothered by the reminder. The pieces of hair are not nearly as bothersome if they are short. If you prefer, you can use the shortest guard and leave little or no hair at all. This is your choice.

How long do I have before my hair starts to fall out?

You may have some warning that you will begin to lose your hair. Many women have told us that they experience head pain a few days prior to the start of their hair loss, like a bad sunburn. It has been explained to me that this is the feeling of the chemotherapy as it is killing the fast growing cells inside the hair follicles. However, the healthy cells are repaired quickly, making your hair loss temporary. You may lose some or all of your hair. According to the MayoClinic.com, hair generally starts falling out one to three weeks after you begin your cancer treatment. It could fall out very quickly, in clumps, or more gradually. Your hair loss could continue throughout your treatment and up to a few weeks after your treatment has stopped. (par. 6, 7)

When my hair falls out, what should I do?

First, even though your hair is gone you should not neglect your scalp. I would recommend washing your scalp with *professional salon shampoo*. The shampoo will remove any impurities and dead skin cells that may accumulate on your scalp and it is gentle. Moisturize your scalp with the same product that you use to moisturize your face.

A stylist I have worked with told me a story about a 74-year-old woman that she had helped to get through her cancer journey. This phenomenal woman found a great way to help keep normalcy in her life during her struggle—she kept her standing weekly appointments with the stylist, just to retain her connection with her salon. She had her head shampooed and massaged, and engaged in her regular conversations with the members of the hair salon staff, as she always had done. This helped her keep a feeling of normalcy about something very important in her life, and she smiled and laughed and enjoyed every moment.

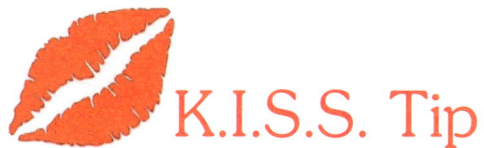

K.I.S.S. Tip

Some health insurance policies cover the cost of a hairpiece needed because of cancer treatment. It is also a tax-deductible expense. Be sure to check your policy and ask your doctor for a "prescription."

> *"I don't consider myself bald. I'm just taller than my hair."*
> – Seneca

Chapter 7

My Hair Is Gone... Now What?

Once you have dealt with the process of hair loss (in whichever way you decide is best for you), there are many ways to cover your head during the time between chemotherapy and when your hair returns. There are women who opt not to use a wig—they do not like the feel of the wig cap, or the seams irritate a radiated area, or it may feel too confining—but I have found that it is not so much about a wig as it is about the *right wig*.

But, besides a wig, there are many other options to conceal your hairless head or just to keep it warm. The choice is up to you.

> **"As long as I can wear a wig I can be any character, and in real life I can be myself."**
>
> – Ginnifer Goodwin

History

According to Wikipedia.com, "the ancient Egyptians wore wigs to shield their shaved, hairless heads from the sun. They also wore the wigs on top of their hair using beeswax and resin to keep the wigs in place. Other ancient cultures…also used wigs as an everyday fashion." The Egyptian people indicated a person's social status as well as their role in society and politics by their wig. Women's wigs were adorned with braids of gold and ivory ornaments, making them more stylish than the men's wigs.

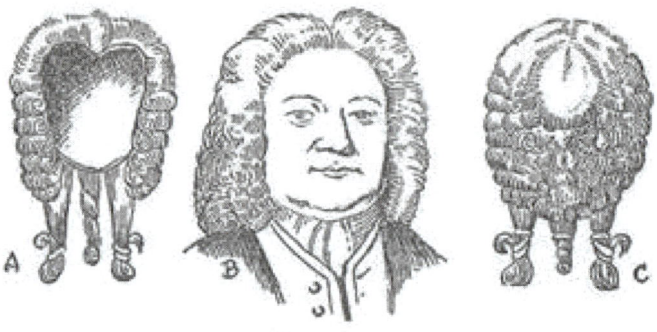

E-Wigs.com. states that "the word 'wigs,' itself, is taken from 'periwigs' which was the name of the particular long, curly wigs that became popular after Charles II was returned to the throne [of England] in 1660." (par. 8) The wig simulated real hair and was primarily used for adornment or to cover the loss of real hair. This style of wig is still used for effect in both the British Parliament and in their judiciary system. Wigs became extremely sought after as they became a symbol of status.

E-Wigs.com also said that "[w]ith the emergence of Christian influences during the medieval era [wigs] became plainer. By the Middle Ages (1200-1400 A.D.) wigs lost their relevance because of difficult times. Women were usually required to have their head covered… Then, in the beginning of [the] Renaissance (1400-1600) the female hairstyle regained importance…" (par. 4) Women's wigs re-emerged because fashion and beauty became important to society once again.

Don't Flip Your Wig!

In my 25+ years as a hairdresser, I cannot tell you the number of times that one of my clients has sat in my chair and confided in me that she has cancer. There were times when I knew before her husband or her family. One of the first things that she would say to me is, "Oh My!! I am going to lose my hair!" Many times this is the first thing that crosses her mind and the first question that she asks the doctor. Hair is very important to us, as women. As I have said before, it is our crowning glory. The correct wig can ease this fear and give a sense of normalcy that is needed, through this all-but-normal time.

Kathy was one of the makeovers that we performed on our six-week tour several years ago. We surprised her while she was shopping in a mall in Muncie, Indiana. She had no clue what was about to happen to/for her. Once the shock of a full day of pampering wore off, I had a chance to speak with Kathy about her wig. She told me that she purchased her wig online by herself, took it out of the box and placed it on her head. No styling, no help. She said it was just "OK" and it camouflaged her bald head as she intended. It did not necessarily flatter her appearance. What I noticed most was that it certainly did not make her feel Gorgeous!

I went to my wig closet in the mobile Day Spa and peeked through our inventory. I found a wig with a spunky style in a similar color and length to Kathy's current wig. I presented the wig to her with no obligation and asked her if she would like to venture into the land of the unknown: a new wig.

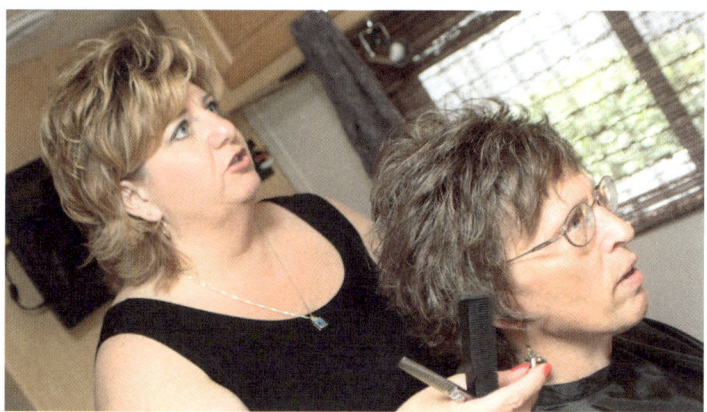

We placed the wig on her head and her face lit up like a Christmas tree. You could see the confidence return, even some spunk and playfulness. It was perfect. We trimmed and styled the wig to flatter Kathy's face shape. It looked as natural as her own hair when we were finished. Mostly, it complemented her personality.

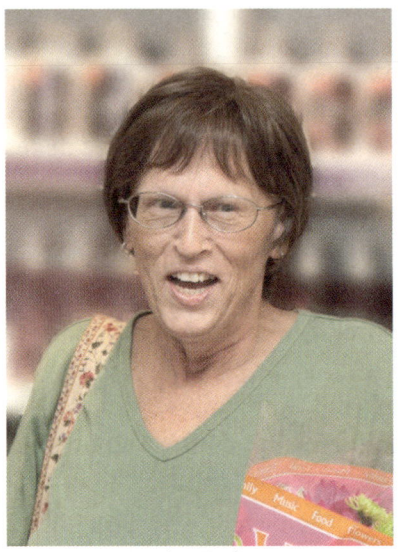
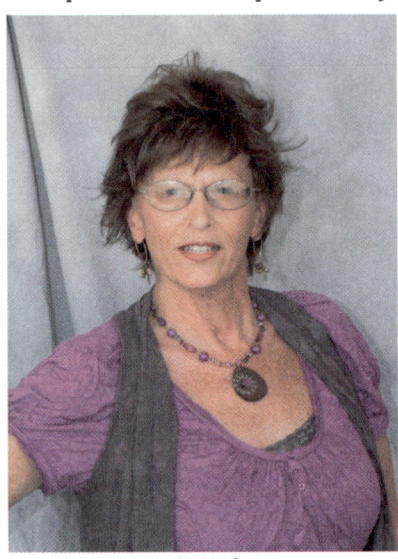

Kathy Before	Kathy After

I know that this is all new to you. More than likely you have never even touched a wig before, let alone know the difference between human hair and synthetic hair, but I am here to help.

But first, let's determine your *face shape*.

How to Determine Your Face Shape

I learned years ago that the perfect face shape is oval. This shape of face can wear any length and any style of hair. This is what I strive for when creating a new style for someone. If your face is not naturally oval, your hair or wig can act as a frame. Like what a picture frame can do for a picture, the shaping of your hair or wig can give you the illusion of an oval-shaped face.

First, let us determine the shape of your face. Stand closely in front of a mirror and, if you do have hair, pull it back and away from your face. With your other hand, trace an outline of your face onto the mirror using something removable (washable marker, lipstick, eyeliner or a bar of soap). Then step back from the mirror and take a look.

Now, we will take a peek at the different face shapes. Please keep in mind that the medication that you are on can alter the natural shape of your face. If it seems fuller than normal, remember that this is most likely temporary. This will help you choose a wig style during your hair loss and a hair style for when you are cancer-free.

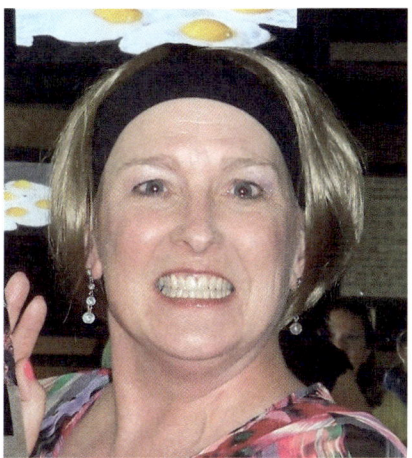
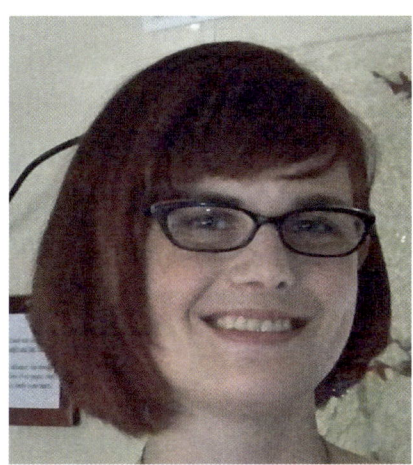

Elaine - Oval Shaped   Isabelle - Round Shaped

Oval-Shaped Face
Your jaw is slightly narrower than your temples and your hairline is gently rounded. With an oval shaped face you can wear most any hairstyle and wear it most any length. Avoid a heavy bang or a style worn toward your face.

Round-Shaped Face
This face shape is wide at the hairline and is full below the cheekbones. An off-center part helps to offset the fullness of a round face. Use the arch of your eyebrow or the highest part of your brow bone to create a part. Creating height in the crown of your head will elongate your face. Avoid chin-length styles, a part down the center of your head and straight-cut heavy bangs. A haircut close to the face is very complementary.

Rectangle-Shaped Face

Rectangle-shaped faces are about 1½ times longer than they are wide. The cheek lines from the temples to the jawline are straight. Adding multiple layers in your hair can open up the cheekbone area and add bulk at the sides of the face. It will give the face shape and balance. You never want extra-long hair if you have a rectangular face and adding a soft, rounded bang can also soften this look.

Heart-Shaped Face

This face shape is wider at the forehead and narrow at the jawline. Try to draw attention to your eyes when choosing a hairstyle or a wig. Short hair looks great on this face shape. A strong part with a side bang is also very complementary. Avoid short, blunt bangs and choppy layers. Keep the hair close to the head around the eye area, but make it slightly fuller around the jawline to create a balance.

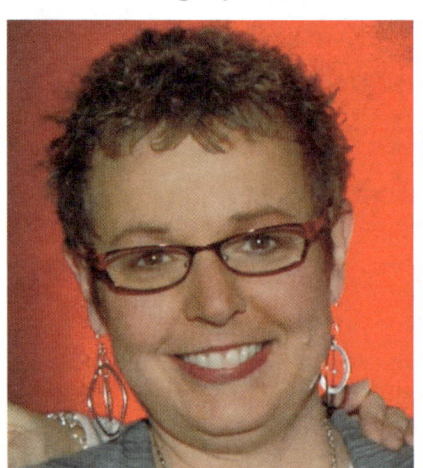
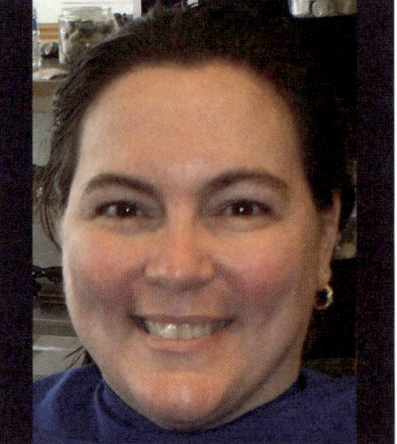

Lynne - Rectangle Shaped   Christina - Heart Shaped

Square-Shaped Face

The width of the face at the forehead, the cheekbones, and the jawline are the same. Your face is nearly as wide as it is long. The hairstyles that are longer with layers that start at the jawline are very complementary. Soft, side-swept bangs that are wispy accentuate the positive features of a square-shaped face. Avoid chin-length bobs and straight-across bangs with this shape of face.

Curly texture and wisps of hair around the face break the wide, straight lines common to this shape.

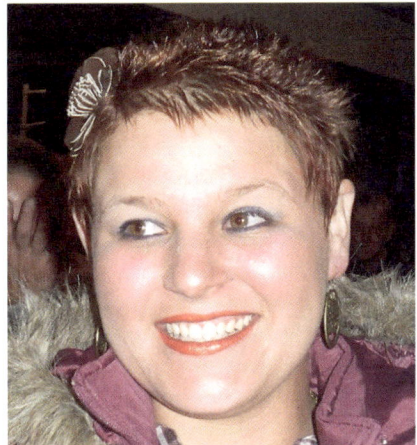
Laura - Square Shaped

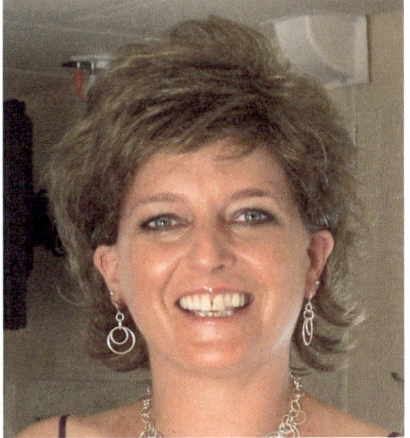
Elise - Diamond Shaped

Diamond-Shaped Face

Your chin will be narrow and pointed. You will also notice high cheekbones and a narrow hairline. Keeping the hair full at the sides with minimum height on the top of the head will complement a diamond-shaped face. Layers that frame your face also work very well. Avoid center parts, heavy straight bangs and short bangs (brow level and above). Also avoid excessive height on the top of the head.

Now that you have your face shape and the best ways to portray your particular look, here are the differences between the types of wigs and how to successfully use them to look your best when you wish to.

Synthetic Hair Wigs

Synthetic wigs are primarily made up of *mod acrylic fibers* that have the look and feel of real hair. These fibers have style memory which allows the original style to be restored. They do not fade in color as can a human-hair wig. These wigs are not porous, which means that they will not absorb odors. With proper care these wigs can last six to nine months.

Synthetic wigs are:
- Very low maintenance;
- CANNOT have a blow dryer, flat iron, or curling iron used on them;
- Tend to be less expensive;
- Bounces back into shape after shampooing;
- Can lack versatility—whatever style it is, is the style that it stays.

(NOTE: I have never had any success changing the style of a synthetic wig. For example, if the part is on the left, it cannot be changed to the right.)

Human Hair Wigs

Human hair wigs are made entirely of human hair and are primarily cut in India and China. Wigs made with human hair are very durable and can last well over a year. However, they require much more maintenance than a synthetic wig. Human-hair wigs must be styled on a regular basis, much like the hair on your head, but they can look and feel more authentic. Human-hair wigs:
- Can be cut and styled as if it were the hair on your head;
- Can have a blow dryer, curling iron, or flat iron used on them;
- Tend to be heavier than a synthetic wig, and more expensive;
- Has to be styled each time the wig is shampooed just as if it were the hair on your head.

How do I put this thing on my head?

Let me walk you through putting your wig on your head, step by step. First, you want to make sure that it fits comfortably and that it is on straight before any assessments are made and before any cutting is done.

1. Look at the inside of your wig. Toward the nape of the wig (or what should be worn against your neck) there should be *an adjuster*. It may be two Velcro tabs or

it may be a series of hooks that fit into ribbon loops. These will help tighten and loosen the fit of your wig.
2. I find the easiest way to place the wig on your head is to find the tabs on the sides of the wig. Many times, they are in the shape of triangles and these triangles will sit in front of your ears. Place your thumbs on the triangles on the inside of the wig. While holding these triangles, turn the wig upside down. Then, in one motion, place the wig the correct way on top of your head (almost like you are holding a bowl and you were going to turn the bowl upside down on your head). Then, pull the wig snugly onto your head.
3. Now adjust the wig, front to back. You want to see your eyes but not your entire forehead. The front of the wig should sit where your hairline used to be. The back of the wig should sit at the base of your head, at the nape of your neck.
4. Adjust the wig from side to side if you need to; but, by placing it on the way you did, it should be correct.
5. How does the wig feel? If it is too tight or too loose, you can remove it and readjust the tabs at the nape of the neck. Then start again at Step 1.

Now take an assessment of your wig

Let's face it: the wig may not look like your own hair. It may not be exact, but we can get it pretty close. In order to do so, you need to take a good look at the wig on your head and ask yourself these questions:
- Where does bulk need to be removed?
- How much fullness needs to be removed? A little or a lot?
- Is the wig too long?
- Where does length need to be removed?
- How much length needs to be removed? A little or a lot?

It would be an ideal situation if you had a professional hairstylist that you trusted. They can help you with this assessment and then take care of any issues you might have. As a woman, I also know that I can be ultra-critical of myself. It is helpful to have an unbiased opinion of your new style from someone you trust. And please always keep in mind that this is *not* forever. This is only temporary, just a season in your life. Your own hair should be back before you know it!

Caring for Your Wig

As I stated earlier, I understand that this may be your first exposure to a wig. It needs to be cared for on a regular basis. Please read the instructions that may have come with your wig. Here are a few steps that can be followed to keep your wig fresh and looking new.

Shampooing instructions for your synthetic wig

1. Give the wig the "Whiff Test."
   (Smell the inside of the wig. That will be the indicator of when it is time to shampoo the wig.)
2. Dampen the wig with lukewarm water.
3. Place a gentle wig shampoo on the inside of the wig cap (the part of the wig that touches your scalp). Wig shampoo is inexpensive and is less harsh than normal shampoo for this use.
4. *Gently* rub the material (inside the wig cap) together to shampoo and squeeze the bubbles into the hair for about 5 minutes.
5. *Do not* rub the hair on the wig. Remember when we were little girls and we thought that it would be fun to give our dolly a bath—and then when we washed her hair, it turned into a matted mess? It will be the same with your wig.
6. Rinse the wig until the water runs clear.
7. Squeeze the water out of the wig.
8. Place the wig in a towel and roll it up, squeezing the excess water from the wig into the towel.
9. Remove the wig from the towel and shake it.
10. Dry the wig by placing it on a 2-liter pop bottle, rather

than the Styrofoam head. This allows the air to flow through the wig cap, which allows your wig to dry more quickly and completely.
11. When the wig is dry, brush or comb into place and style as usual.

(NOTE: Do not place the wig on the foam head while it is wet, as it may stretch it out. In addition, do not attempt to comb or brush the wig when it is wet.)

Shampooing instructions for your human hair wig
1. Give wig the "Whiff Test."
2. Remove tangles with comb, brush or pick prior to shampooing.
3. Dampen wig with lukewarm water.
4. Place a gentle shampoo on the inside of the wig cap
5. Gently rub the material together to shampoo and squeeze the bubbles into the hair, about 5 minutes.
6. Rinse until the water runs clear.
7. Apply a small amount of conditioner and massage into the wig. Rinse well with lukewarm water.
8. Place the wig in a towel and roll it up, squeezing the excess water from the wig into the towel.
9. Remove the wig from the towel and shake it.
10. Comb or brush wig to remove the tangles and comb into shape.
11. Place the wig on a 2-liter pop bottle to dry. You can also dry a human hair wig with a blow dryer set on low heat and low speed.
12. Comb or brush the wig gently. Style your human hair wig using hot rollers or curling iron. Set the wig with a wig spray or a light hairspray.

How to maintain a healthy scalp under your wig
It is important to take care of your scalp with or without hair. Here are a few steps to help maintain a healthy scalp under your wig. These steps will help to avoid:

- Dandruff
- Formation of Bacteria
- Further hair loss, thinning hair, and/or breakage of existing hair

1. Wash your scalp regularly using a *professional salon shampoo*. Again, inexpensive drugstore shampoos are full of waxes and plastics that can build up on your scalp and inhibit the growth of new hair.
2. Make certain that, if you do have some hair, you never leave it wet under your wig. Always dry your hair and scalp prior to placing your wig on your head.
3. Moisturize your scalp using the same moisturizer that you use on your face.
4. Let your scalp breath. Just as if it were a hat, remove your wig every night before going to sleep.
5. Be sure to use a good sunscreen if you go out without an adequate head covering. Some of this skin has not experienced full sun since you were an infant!

Removable Bangs

I love these things. My mother-in-law, Jeanine, had a brain tumor and, because of where the radiation took place, it was very difficult for her to wear a wig. The wig was resting on the radiation burn and it was extremely uncomfortable for her. The radiation burn also itched. This is not even talking about the staples in her scalp from the surgery. So we needed to come up with an alternative to a wig. We opted for a terrycloth turban, which is soft to the touch and had some removable bangs.

A *removable bang* is hair that is attached to a Velcro strip or connected to a headband and these can easily be worn under or attached to a turban, hat or scarf. The bangs can come in various widths. They can also range in lengths and colors. The whole assembly is reasonably priced. These removable bangs can also be personalized by your stylist. Your stylist can trim them and texturize them to create the perfect look for you.

You can find these and other amazing tools at your local boutique that specializes in hair-loss items. Your hospital or doctor's office should be able to direct you to the nearest boutique of this type.

Cold Head at Night

Here is something you may not have thought of. During this time when you have little or no hair (maybe for the first time in your life), your scalp is exposed and your head can get cold, especially at night. You may want to invest in a nightcap—a loose-fitting cotton hat that you can wear to bed at night. If you don't want to spend the money, there is an inexpensive solution to keep your head warm.

Take an old t-shirt, long or short sleeve, and cut the sleeves off at the seam from the armpit to the shoulder. This makes a perfect nightcap and the material is soft and soothing to the soft tissue of your scalp. Easy!

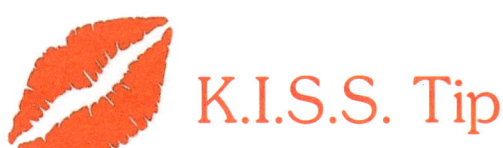 K.I.S.S. Tip

Dry off your head with a clean dry towel. Squirt a pea-sized amount of a non-alcohol-based moisturizer on your head. Spread it all over your scalp from front to back with your hands. Let the moisturizer dry for 10 minutes. Apply a gentle, non-irritating sunscreen to your head the same way as the moisturizer. Sunscreen prevents sunburn on your head, which leads to peeling and drying.

Alternative Head Coverings

SCARVES

A scarf, by definition, is a length of fabric that is worn around the head or neck. There are many reasons that women wear headscarves. Some women wear them as a fashion statement, to add color to an outfit or to perk up an otherwise boring hairstyle. Some women wear headscarves for religious beliefs. According to USCAnnenberg, "Headscarves actually accentuate many women's beauty by drawing attention to the face and away from the hair and the body. In many cultures, the face is more important as a place of beauty than is the body, and head-covers facilitate this focus toward the face, facial expression, conversation, etc...." (par. 9) I would have to assume that, if you are reading this book, your reason for needing a head covering is due to your cancer treatment.

Here are a few alternatives to your wig that can look cute and fashionable while serving the purpose of *camouflaging* your hairless head. Scarves can be a wonderful alternative for covering your head while going through cancer treatment and dealing with hair loss. Natural fabrics, for example 100-percent cotton, work best. They are less likely to slip off your head and the cotton prevents excess perspiration. It also is more comfortable against your scalp.

Have fun when choosing the fabric for your scarves. Choose bright vibrant colors, colors that look good on you (refer to the colors explanation in the fashion chapter of this book). Choose patterns that make you smile. Keep in mind that this is not forever; it is just a means to an end—to get you healthy.

Here are (4) Scarf-Folding Techniques:

Back-knot scarf

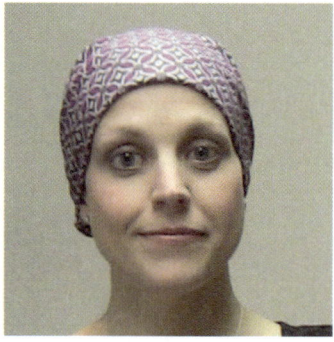
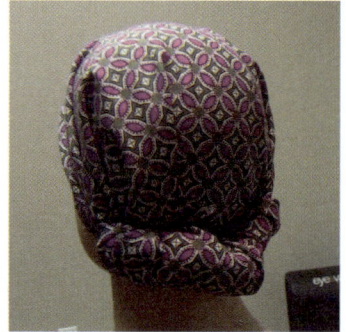

My Hair is Gone...Now What? < 75

Begin with a piece of fabric that is between 30- and 36-inches square, depending on the size of your head. Lay the fabric flat on the table, pattern-side down, so it looks like a square.

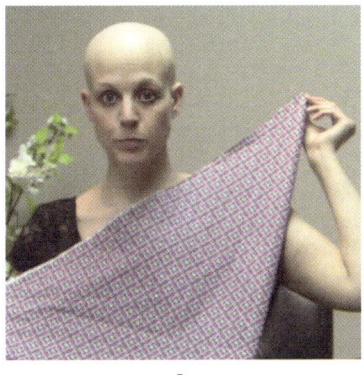
1

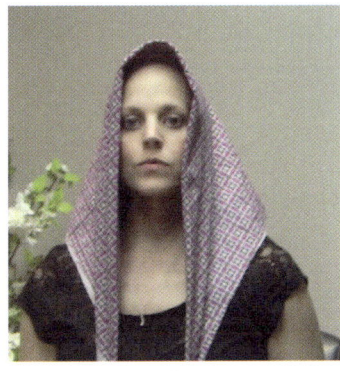
2

1) Fold the scarf diagonally to make a triangle, corner to corner.

2) Pick up your triangle, placing the center of the longest straight edge of your triangle on your forehead at the hairline. You should have one point by each ear and one point of the triangle at the back of your head. The triangle should be covering your entire head.

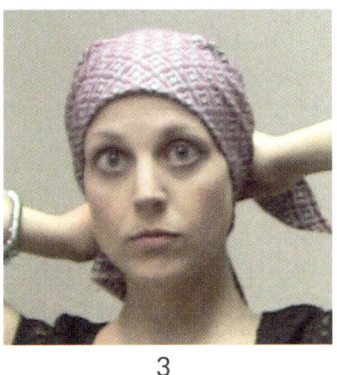
3

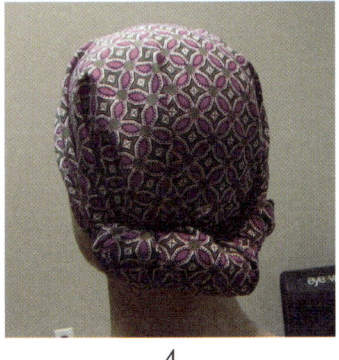
4

3) Pick up the points of the triangle at each ear, one in each hand, and then tie them together at the back of your head, leaving the third point loose.

4) You can fold the third point (that lies against your neck) over the knot that you just created in the back of your head and then tuck it underneath the knot of the scarf to hide it, to create a smooth finished look.

Turban Headscarf

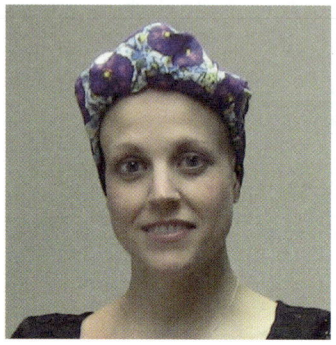
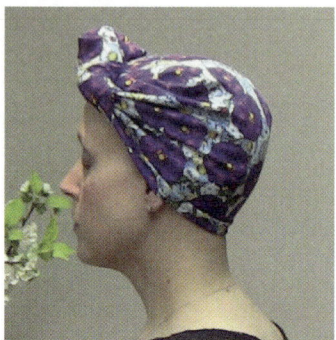

Begin with a piece of fabric that is between 30- and 36-inches square, depending on the size of your head. Lay the fabric flat on the table, pattern-side down, so it looks like a square.

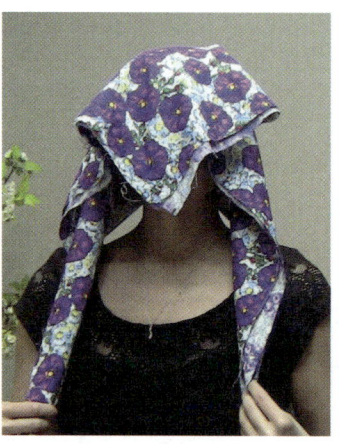
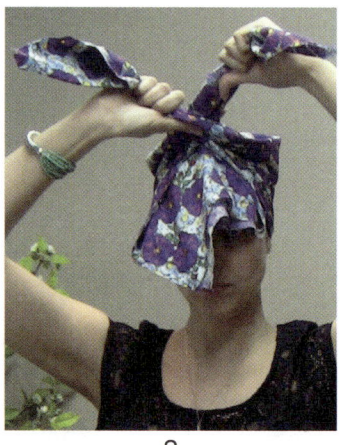

1   2

1) Pick up the triangle and place the center of the longest straight edge at the back of your head (just below the base of the skull). You should have one point on your forehead, hanging past the bridge of your nose, and one point at each ear.

2) Now take the points by your ears, one in each hand, and pull the ends up and forward, past your face, and tie the ends into a knot at your forehead.

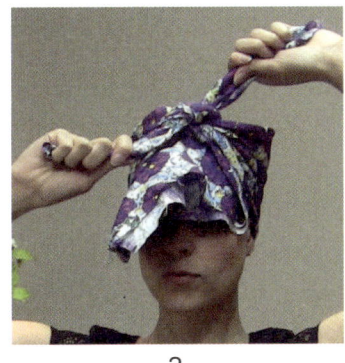
3

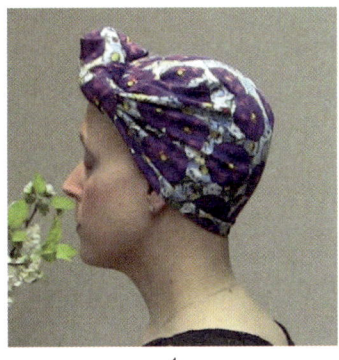
4

3) Tuck the ends of the two points under the knot that you just made.

4) You can fold the third point (that hangs over your face) over the knot that you just created on your forehead and then tuck the end underneath the inside of the knot to hide it, to create a smooth finished look.

Side-rose Scarf

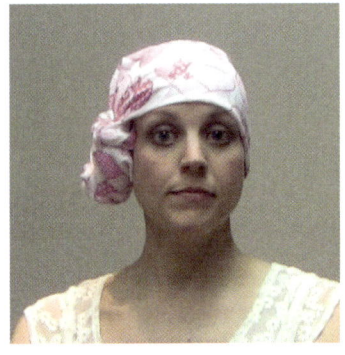
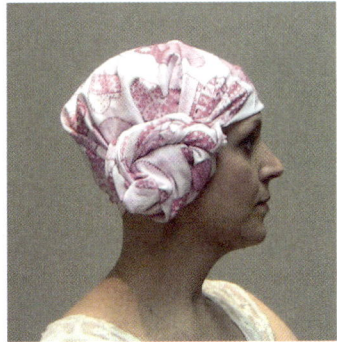

Begin with a piece of fabric that is between 30- and 36-inches square, depending on the size of your head. Lay the fabric flat on the table, pattern-side down, so it looks like a square.

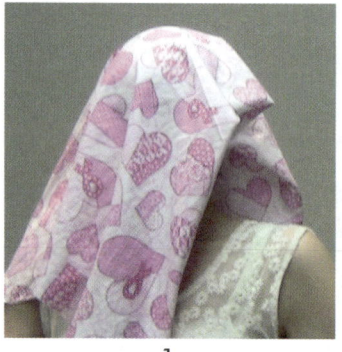 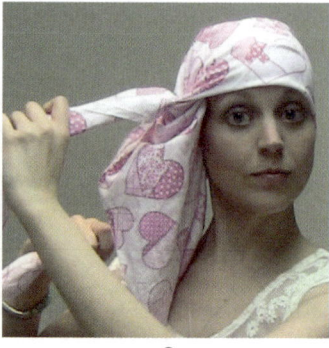

1   2

1) Place the long, straight edge of the scarf and center it over your left or right ear, dependent on where you want the "rose." You should have one point in front of your face, one at the back of your head and the tail over your right ear.

2) Bring both ends together around your head, at the side of one ear, and tie them into a knot.

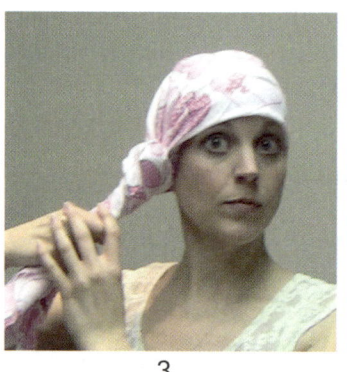 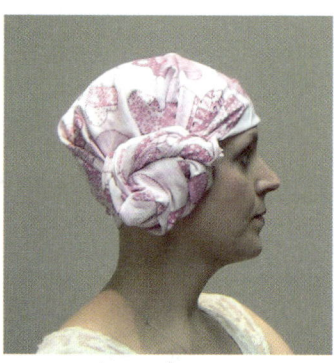

3   4

3) Make sure that the front and back create smooth edges along your forehead and neck.

4) Take all three ends into one hand and twist them tightly, circling them into a knot against your ear to form a rosette. Tuck the end under the rosette to secure it into place.

A rope wrap

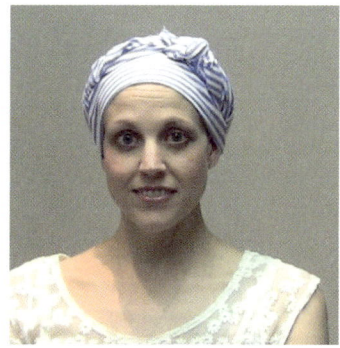 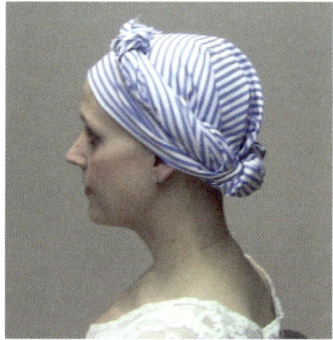

Begin with a piece of fabric that is between 30- and 36-inches square, depending on the size of your head. Lay the fabric flat on the table, pattern-side down, so it looks like a square.

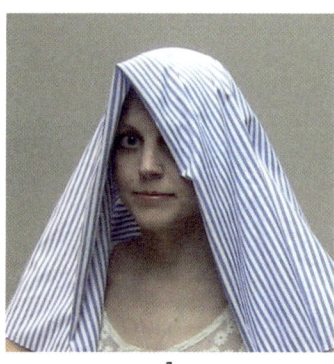 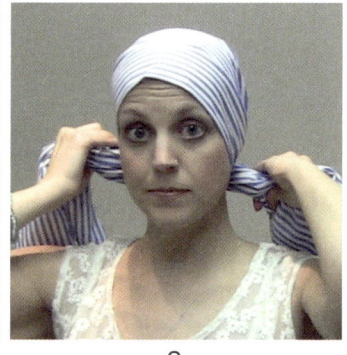

1   2

1) Drape the scarf over your head. Make sure that the scarf is evenly centered and that one of the longest edges is sitting on your forehead.

2) Gather the end of the scarves in each hand, at ear level, on the sides of your head. Move them back to the nape of the neck and cross them behind your head and pull tightly.

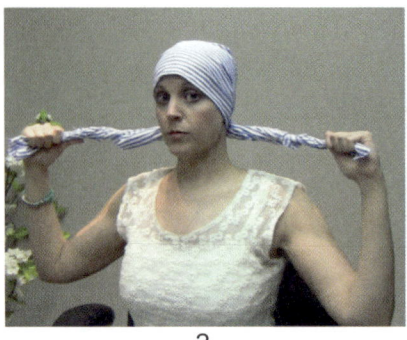 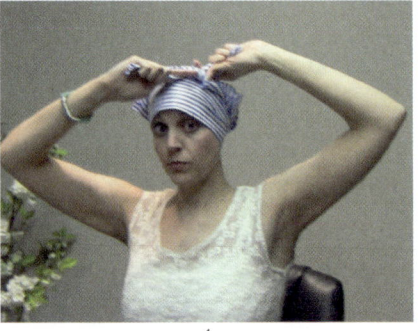

3   4

3) Form a rope by twisting the scarf. You should have one end of the scarf in each hand.

4) Bring the twisted ends of the scarf around and up to your forehead. If the ends are short, tie them at the forehead and tuck the ends under the knot to give a finish look.

If the ends are long enough, cross the ropes at the forehead as well and wrap them around toward the back, following the shape of your head. Tie a knot at the nape of the neck or tuck the ends under the knot to finish the look.

Hats, Hats, Hats

A great majority of you have never before worn a hat. Here is a very useful tool for making the choice of a correct hat a bit easier. It is the *Hat Wearing Guide for Cancer Chemotherapy Patients* from HeadCovers.com :

- Look for deep hats that fit down over your head in the 1920s style. Cloth ones work very well.
  Men's-style hats, like an Annie Hall look, can also be very complementary.
- Avoid hats that you can see through. They most likely will not hide your hair loss nor protect you from the sun.
- Think about where you would be wearing your hat. Wide brims can be fun outdoors and do a great job blocking UV rays.

Consider your overall shape

- Your hat should not be any wider than the width of your shoulders.
- If you are petite, you should choose a hat with a low-profile crown and a small brim. Avoid big hats that can overpower you.
- If you are tall, hats with a wide brim and a short crown are the most flattering. Stay away from narrow and angular-shaped hats.
- If you are full figured, hats with a wide, full brim can balance your shape.

Consider your face shape

- If you have a long face, hats with a wide, flat brim or a curled, floppy brim work well. Try pulling the brim of your hat down to your eyebrow to shorten your face. Avoid hats with narrow brims and hats that are tall. These can add length to you face.
- If you have a round or square face, select hats with a high brim and asymmetrical shapes. Avoid round, circular or floppy-shaped hats. Wear your brims on an angle whenever possible. The crown of your hat should be at least as wide as your face.
- If you have a heart-shaped face, you should look for hats with asymmetric shapes.
- If you have an oval or triangular-shaped face, you can wear almost any style of hat. Make sure that the crown is never narrower than your cheekbones.

Consider the position of the hat

- If a hat isn't flattering when you first try it on, you may need to adjust how it is sitting on your head. You may not be wearing it far enough forward or back. Angle it to its best advantage—maybe tilting it slightly to the right or the left. Angle it from *every* direction and look at it from *every* angle. Experiment until you find the best look for you.

Consider accessories

- If you wear glasses, try up turning the brim of your hat up for a more flattering look.
- If you have hair, try tucking your hair behind your ears or putting your hair up. Whatever you are comfortable with will be the best look for you.
- Experiment with different earrings to add interest.
- Scarves are a wonderful way to give a very classy look to a very plain hat. Tie a scarf around the perimeter of the hat and it will dress it up just like that. You can also color coordinate the scarf with whichever outfit you may be wearing that day.

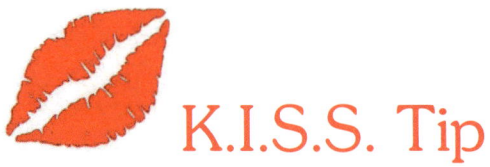 K.I.S.S. Tip

Choose a hat that suits your face and frame. If you've got a big jawline, for example, a cowboy hat can help balance it out with that wider brim. But if you're petite, it might overwhelm you. Shop around for the right look!

"It doesn't matter who you are, or where you came from. The ability to triumph begins with you. Always."

– Oprah Winfrey

Chapter 8

My Hair Has Stayed, But It's Not the Same

Chemotherapy can wreak havoc on your hair, even if it does not always make it fall out. Cancers that use solely radiation therapy will cause you to lose hair only in the radiated areas. But these still can cause changes to your hair and scalp normalcy.

Here are a few suggestions to help in these areas.

"The only way to make sense out of change is to plunge into it, move with it, and join the dance."

– Alan Watts

Cha-Cha-Changes!

As I understand it, all hair on the body can be affected by chemotherapy. Experts in this area say that, when you stop your chemotherapy, it is very common for the hair to grow back differently.

"We don't know how chemotherapy affects the cell cycle," says Dr. Doris Day, a board-certified dermatologist and clinical assistant professor of dermatology at NYU Medical Center, and author of the book *Forget the Facelift* (Avery Penguin, 2008). "But the thing is that chemotherapy does seem to affect the hair cycle. After chemotherapy, the hair may start cycling differently."

Strange things can happen: straight hair may go curly, or curly hair straight; gray hair may go dark again, or (many times) dark hair goes gray. In rare cases, it may not grow back at all. It can be thinner all around, or thin in only some areas—like male-pattern baldness. Sometimes, the hair reverts to its original color and texture after a year or two. Sometimes, it doesn't.

There is no way to know how chemotherapy will impact your hair until it actually grows back. But here are some suggestions to help you cope with the changes that may take place in your hair during your cancer treatment.

Dry or Brittle Hair from Treatment

1. During this time, if you don't need to shampoo your hair every day, then I would recommend not doing so. Keeping some of your own natural oils on your hair can make it feel less brittle.

2. I would suggest conditioning your hair every time you shampoo with a daily conditioner recommended by your salon specialist.

3. You may also use a deep conditioner one to two times a week. Consult your salon specialist, who will recommend the correct product for your hair, and then follow the manufacturer's instructions. I would stay away from conditioners that claim to have protein in them as that can make the hair even more brittle.

4. Sleeping on a satin pillowcase is better for your hair than sleeping on rougher fabrics because the smooth material helps prevent tangles and breakage, as your hair does not get caught on the fabric.

Thinning Hair from Treatment

1. If your cancer treatment thins your hair, one consideration may be to cut your hair shorter than you would normally wear it. This can help give the illusion that there is more there than actually exists. Also, remember to use sunscreen on areas where hair is very thin or gone altogether.

2. There are products out there that will encourage new hair growth. These products are wonderful and I have had some amazing results, but I would not recommend using them until you complete your treatment. On the other hand, there are *professional shampoos, conditioners, mousse and other volumizing products* that *may* be purchased. These will add needed body and volume to your hair to help give you the fullness that you desire.

3. I know you want to hang on to as much hair as possible, but having it trimmed and shaped every four to six weeks will keep your hair manageable for you and it will keep it looking healthy.

4. Remember that this is *not* forever. Ninety percent of the time, once treatment has ended your hair slowly but surely returns to a normal state. But it is *not* immediate. It takes time. Your hair grows approximately ½ inch each month. So in six months' time, your hair should grow about three inches.

Hair Changing Color from Treatment

We have seen a few instances where the hair remains on the head during treatment but it changes color. In one particular case the natural color was a level-6 brown, and the hair lightened to a level-7 and turned an orangey color. If this has happened to you and you do not like the new color that your treatment has blessed you with, this can be helped. Your hair can be colored! Again, I would recommend that this be done by your *professional stylist in the salon*. First, I would request a *patch test*. This is done by applying the color that will be used during your service to the inside of your arm where it bends or behind the ear. Let the color sit for the processing time, usually 30 minutes. Gently remove the color and wait 24 hours to make sure that no redness or itching occurs. If no reaction occurs, you can proceed with the color service. When you go to the salon, explain to the stylist what you are going through and show them what has happened. If you have a picture of yourself when you loved the color of your hair, take that picture with you. Ask your stylist to perform a *strand test* to see what your hair will do when color is applied to it.

A *strand test* is where a small amount of the desired color is mixed up by your stylist and placed on a small section of your hair, and left there for the full processing time. The color is then removed with a towel and checked against the intended color, to make sure that you have achieved the desired results. Remember that your hair is chemically altered (due to your cancer treatment) so we want to test the waters before we apply the color to your entire head. Once the result is acceptable, proceed with the normal application to the entire head. Process the color according to the manufacturer's instructions. Your stylist will know what to do. Then style your hair as usual.

Salon vs Over-the-Counter Products

Let's talk hair product. Again, I would recommend that you *avoid* using products on your hair that are not purchased at a salon. Many products for your hair found in drugstores or grocery stores have additives like plastic, waxes and high amounts of alcohol. The plastic and waxes in these products are not water soluble and, over a long period of time, may build up on your hair and scalp, which may slow the re-growing process. These products can also weigh your hair down and give it an oily appearance. This in turn may cause you to shampoo your hair more often, which can be drying to the hair.

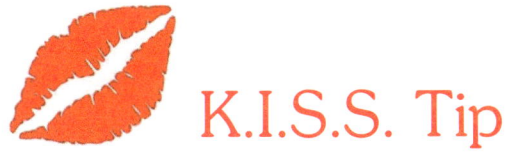

K.I.S.S. Tip

Your makeup will always look better when applied to a clean, moisturized face!

> ***"You are altogether beautiful, my love;***
> ***There is no flaw in you."***
>
> – Song of Solomon 4:7

Chapter 9

My Hair Grew Back... Now What?

These are exciting times when, after weeks and months of waiting, you are past your chemotherapy—you look in the mirror and see the first hint of hair sprouting from your scalp! We know you are fiercely proud of this hair, and we can help you make your short hair look deliberate and fabulous! Here we go!

> *"I was going to buy a book on hair loss, but the pages kept falling out!"*
> – Jay London

Laura's Story

Laura was a young girl who had to grow up very fast. She was 24 years old when we met her and she had already been diagnosed with a very aggressive form of breast cancer. She had 24 hours to make a decision concerning having a double mastectomy. She had two children under the age of four and, during all of this, her husband made the decision that all of this was too much for him to handle, so he left Laura and the children to seek a divorce.

When we surprised Laura with a makeover, we found that Laura was a tiny, petite thing wearing this huge, dark "Loretta Lynn"-style wig. It was very overpowering on her but, once we got her into the mobile DaySpa and she took off that monstrous wig, we found that she had about 4 beautiful inches of her own hair under it. It was certainly enough to work with. So, our team of experts went to work and performed their magic on Laura. We cut and colored her new hair and gave her some hints and tips on how to style it. When we finished, she looked adorable and sported her new look into her Reveal Party with gusto!

As my husband Mike escorted her into the restaurant, he asked her how she felt. Laura said, "I wish my ex-husband could see me now!" You could tell that she felt good about herself—especially her hair. It was like watching a butterfly emerge from a cocoon.

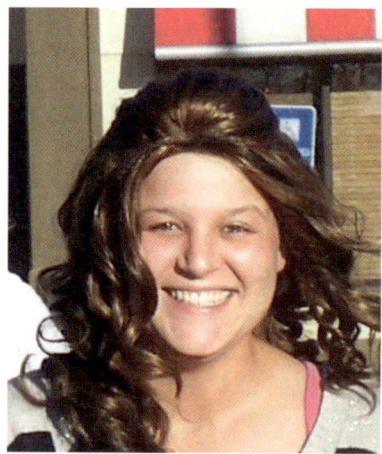
Laura Before

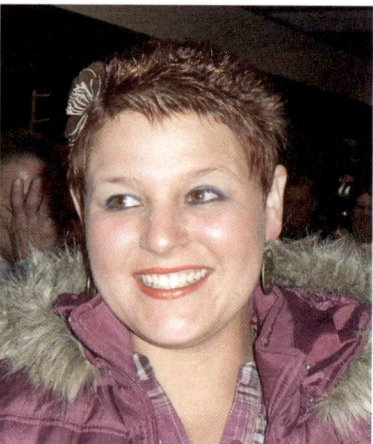
Laura After

Make It Look Deliberate

Losing your hair as a woman can be devastating. This is our crowning glory! It is sometimes the first thing you *see* when you look in the mirror. Consequently, it is also the first thing you notice is missing after it all falls out through chemo. But the good news is that 90% of the time it grows back! As I mentioned earlier, your hair grows a half an inch per month on average. It may take a few months after chemotherapy treatment to *see* substantial growth but, once you are able to place your hand flat on your scalp and pinch hair between your second and middle finger, it is time to get a haircut. Yes, I *know* you just got it back—after a long time without *any* hair—and I know that you do not want to part with *any* of it. But believe me when I tell you that it will look much better if you have it trimmed at this point. Removing those little fuzzy ends can make a huge difference. I always tell my clients that at this point we can shape your hair and make it look *deliberate*—like you have always wanted your hair short and you had it cut short on purpose—not like someone who just finished cancer treatment. It will amaze you what a difference an eighth of an inch can make! So...

1. Don't be afraid;
2. Go to someone you trust who will listen to you;
3. Remember that professional styling products will be your best friend.

Changes? We Can Help!

Again, when your hair grows back after chemotherapy you may notice some differences, compared to the hair you had before you lost it. It may now be:

- More curly;
- More gray;
- A completely different color or texture.

Once your stylist shapes your hair, she can suggest some styling aids that will help you with your style. Here are some suggestions:

Mousse

Mousse is applied to towel-dried hair. A golf ball-sized portion should be plenty of product. Put the product in the palm of one hand, rub your palms together to get the product equally on both hands and place the hands on your head to evenly distribute the mousse throughout your hair. Then style as directed by your stylist.

Wax, pomade, paste, or putty

After your hair is blown dry, place a small amount of wax, pomade, paste, or putty (about the size of a pea) in the palm of one hand. Rub your hands together to distribute the product evenly. Place your hands in your hair and squeeze your hair between your fingers. This will apply the perfect amount of product evenly through your hair and will make it look separated, more modern and deliberate.

Gel

I would use a gel if you need control and not volume. If your hair has grown back wiry or extremely curly, gel will give you the most control. Gel has a tendency to be heavy and slick down the hair shaft, so use it sparingly.

Hairspray

When you are happy with the way that your hair looks, you can finish your style by spraying it into place. You can use an aerosol or a pump hairspray. An aerosol is a drier product and a pump will have more of a moist feel, but it dries as it reaches the hair. Hold the hairspray about 12 inches away from your head and spray just what you need to hold your style. You can spray a small amount of hairspray on your thumb and index finger and pinch the hair around your face, from your bangs to the hair around your ears. This will create some nice framing around your face that will stay and give your new do some added style.

Hair Color

We have done hundreds and hundreds of makeovers and performed a countless number of color services on women who are coming out of treatment with no problems. But I would like to make a few *strong* suggestions:

1. *Do not try this at home.* Your hair and your body have been through a lot of chemical changes. Things are different now—your favorite chestnut brown may end

up "Elvira" black. Leave this to the professionals. Make an appointment at a reputable, local salon.

2. Have a *patch test* done prior to any color service. Again, your body has been through many changes and your body has chemicals in it that it has never seen before. A patch test is easy and will give you peace of mind. When you schedule your color service with your salon, ask them to schedule a patch test. This takes about five minutes. A small amount of the color that will be used at your appointment is mixed up and placed either behind your ear or on the inside of your arm where it bends. This will stay on your skin for 30 minutes and then it is removed and a 24-hour waiting period begins. When you return to the salon for your scheduled service, the salon professional will check the location where the color was placed to make sure that there is no redness or irritation. As long as everything is clear, you may proceed with the color service. Most of the women we have tested came out perfectly, but we have had about five percent who had a reaction. Better just a small spot on your arm or behind your ear than across your entire head!

3. Hair color is a great way to enhance your new short "do." You can add highlights, cover the new gray that was not there before, or simply return to your normal hair color. My opinion—GO FOR IT! Your hair may be shorter than it has *ever* been, so now is the time to have some fun! You made it! You are still here!

I have always heard that blondes have more fun—try it!

If you have heard that redheads have *even more* fun (they just don't talk about it), then Go Red! Have a blast! Change it up!

The Difference between Hair Color and Highlights

First, I want to help you better understand the difference between "on-the-scalp" color and highlights. Remember that knowledge is power. This will help you move forward when deciding on a *deliberate* look with your new hair.

Scalp-to-Ends Color (All-Over Color)

Scalp-to-ends color is applied to the entire head, from your scalp to the ends of your hair. Every single hair on your head will have color applied to it. It can be applied with a bottle or brush.

New Growth Touch-Up

A touch-up is color applied only to the hair that has newly grown in, next to the scalp. A touch-up used to be referred to as "getting your roots done," which is a misnomer since you cannot actually have the roots of your hair colored. This hair is your natural hair color and is free of artificial color as it grows. Again, dependent upon the line of professional color used, it can be applied with a bottle or brush and needs to be redone every four to six weeks.

Highlights

When hair is highlighted, the color is kept off the scalp. Not every hair is colored; so, if you have gray hair, there may still be some present at the end of the color service. Highlights need to be revisited only every 12 to 16 weeks, depending on the contrast of the highlight color(s) to your natural hair color.

The color(s) can be applied to the hair by placing a highlight paper or foil under the hair strands and folding it in, or by pulling it through a cap. If foil or papers are used, multiple colors may be used to create either a soft, natural look or a bold, modern look.

Types of Hair Color Product

Permanent Hair Color

This chemical allows color to penetrate existing strands of hair and infuse them with color. It is designed to cover your existing hair shade and appear as a completely different color, with none of the previous color showing through. This color will grow out—and away from the scalp—as your hair grows (and the new hair growth will be your natural hair color), but it does not wash out, and it will need to be re-colored every four to six weeks to maintain a uniform look.

Demi-Permanent Hair Color

Demi-permanent hair coloring dye is applied to the hair shaft and penetrates between the first and second outermost layers of hair. Demi-permanent color can lighten your natural hair color, deposit rich tones of color and temporarily cover gray hair. It does not last as long as permanent color, so more touch-ups would be needed to hide gray hairs.

Semi-Permanent Hair Color

Semi-permanent hair color is more like a stain. It covers the hair shafts but does not adhere to your hair like a permanent color, so it may not cover the gray as well. Semi-permanent hair color may create more of a gray "blending."

Imagine that you have a piece of wood. When the wood is stained, the grain of the wood is still noticeable but the color of the wood is changed. Semi-permanent color can wash off in four to six weeks and it is non-committal. You can choose never to color again, since the signs of existing color are very faint.

So, now that you have an idea of what kind of hair color you may want to try, and how it can be applied to get your desired effect, you need to decide if you want a color that is subtle, BOLD, or somewhere in between.

Here is an easy way to decide for yourself the best approach for you, and it's an easy way to communicate your wish to your stylist as well.

Hair Color that Whispers, Talks, or Shouts!

As a salon owner, part of my job was to train new stylists who were coming out of beauty school. I wanted these "new talents" to strive to be better stylists than I *ever* was. I informed them that

50% of their job was to first be a detective: to ask questions and to use pictures of different hairstyles during the consultations to make sure that they *understood* exactly what their clients desired so they could *deliver* just that. Color is always one of the toughest services because you need to make sure you achieve the correct tone and the right amount of color. So, I developed a method to help aid in the process. The new talent was coached to ask their client if they wanted their color to whisper, talk, or shout. Even though your stylist may not have been trained in my system, this is a great communication tool to use when consulting about your new color look.

+ To *WHISPER* meant that it is an introduction to color. There will be *subtle* differences, but the client really does not want to draw attention to the fact that they have even participated in a color service.

+ If they want their color to *TALK*, we know that they want it to be more *noticeable*, but not overpowering. They want people to say, "What did you do different?"—but not necessarily ask if they had color done.

+ But, if the client wants their color to *SHOUT*, then we know to pull out all the stops! These clients want people to stop them on the street because they noticed the color!

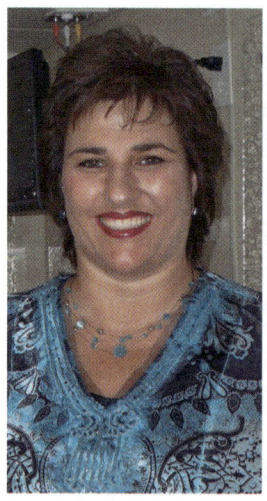
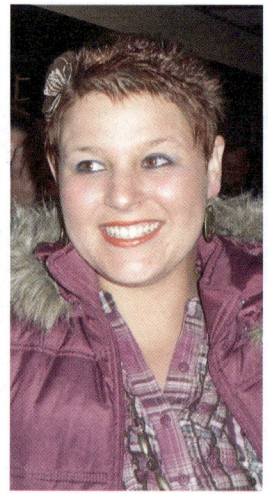
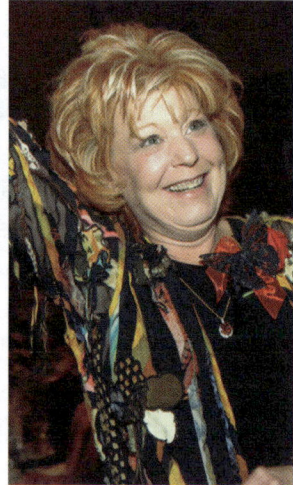

Whisper   Talk   Shout!

Hair Care for Women of Color

Chemotherapy, as we have said before, generally targets all of the fast-growing cells in the body. It does not care what sex, race, or age you are. However, there are different hair textures and different ways of caring for them. This can be important when it comes to the difference between Caucasian hair and African-American hair.

As with all women, your hair may or may not fall out during your cancer treatment. It really depends on your course of treatment and the type of chemotherapy you are given. If you do lose your hair, when it does grow back in, it may also be quite different from your pre-cancer-diagnosis hair. It may be:

- More curly
- More course
- More fine
- Thinner, or
- More gray

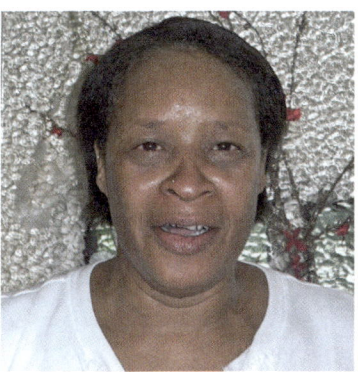
Tanya Before

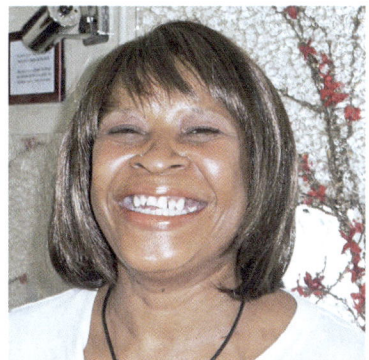
Tanya After

Taking Care of Fragile Hair

African-American hair is more fragile than other textures of hair and more susceptible to breakage. When combing or brushing your new hair, use a wide-tooth comb or a brush with wide, soft, plastic bristles. Avoid hard boar bristle brushes or fine tooth combs.

I would recommend washing your hair weekly, not daily. Curly African-American hair tends to be drier and less oily than European hair, so it requires fewer washings. Avoid products with petroleum, which can make your hair dry, greasy, and stiff. Instead, try natural oils—like coconut, jojoba, olive, or castor oils. These oils will also be good for your scalp as your hair grows back.

Products with natural ingredients such as almond oil will help seal the hair cuticle. Grape seed oil is very light and can withstand high temperatures without scorching. This can be helpful in controlling heat damage if you use heated styling tools.

As your hair is growing back, it will be helpful to sleep on a *silk pillowcase* or sleep with a *silk scarf* around your head. This will help to keep your hair healthy and it will not induce breakage or tearing of the hair follicles while you sleep as your hair is growing back. A cotton pillowcase tends to draw the moisture out of your hair while you sleep, as will a cotton scarf or turban.

Chemical Services

I recommend that hair color or relaxers be applied by a professional stylist to ensure that they are applied safely and to minimize damage to your new hair. My recommendation is to wait at least three months after treatment for hair color, and six months to one year before attempting a relaxer or a perm. First of all, you need to have hair to relax. Second, this will give your body time to adjust to all the chemical changes it has been through. I would also recommend a patch test before attempting any chemical service, and I would have the service performed at a salon by a professional, licensed stylist.

Patch Test

Again, a patch test uses a small amount of the chemical that will be used during the service. It is placed on the inside of your arm or just behind your ear. This is left on the skin for 30 minutes and removed. A waiting period of 24 hours is needed before re-examining the area where the chemical was applied. As long as there is NO redness or irritation, and the stylist thinks that your hair is strong enough to withstand the chemical service, you may proceed. Make sure that the stylist follows the manufacturer's instructions.

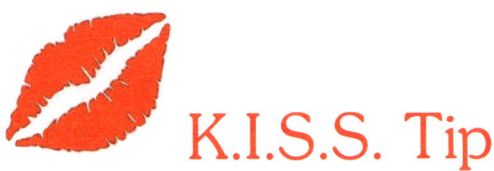 ## K.I.S.S. Tip

If God didn't want you to change your hair, He wouldn't have made it grow!

> ***"If they ever do my life story, whoever plays me needs lots of hair color and high heels."***
>
> – Charlize Theron

Chapter 10

Put Your Best Face Forward

Makeup is one of the most effective weapons in your arsenal for looking Gorgeous! This chapter touches on every category of cosmetics: the right mascara, complimentary blush and eye shadow colors, foundations and concealers, and how to use all of them.

So, get ready to be Gorgeous in any situation!

"People will stare. Make it worth their while."
– Harry Winston

History

Wikipedia states that the first applications of makeup can be traced back to the ancient Egyptians around 4000 B.C. Scientists know this by the contents of their tombs. A simple cosmetic was designed to darken the area around the eyes and was even thought to improve eyesight. "Archaeological evidence of cosmetics certainly dates from ancient Egypt and Greece. According to one source, early major developments include the use of castor oil in ancient Egypt as a protective balm and skin creams made of beeswax, olive oil, and rosewater described by the Romans. The Ancient Greeks also used cosmetics.

"Cosmetics are mentioned in the Old Testament—2 Kings 9:30 where Jezebel painted her eyelids—approximately 840 B.C.—and the book of Esther describes various beauty treatments as well. Cosmetics were also used in ancient Rome, although much of Roman literature suggests that it was frowned upon."

Makeup is found in the history of every major culture in history.

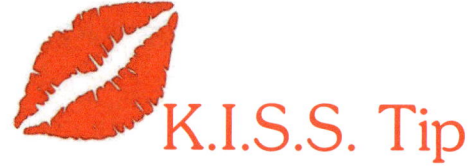

K.I.S.S. Tip

By not removing your makeup nightly it will age your skin by 7 years.

Tina's Story

I have three sisters. Tina, my middle sister, was diagnosed with cancer during the summer of 2012. One of the hardest things I ever had to do was to shave my sister's head—once the chemotherapy kicked in and made it fall out. Two days later, she needed to pick up a prescription from the store, so she just put a hat on and went. During her visit she must have received some stares or looks of pity from some of the other customers.

She texted me from the store and said: *"Why do people look at sick people this way? I hate this!"*

This is a day I will never forget. Luckily I was not helpless. I grabbed my other sister, Trish, who is also a hairdresser and we went to work picking out new makeup for Tina. We stopped at an accessory store, bought her some new bigger earrings, and we cornered her at the house of our other sister, Amy, and ambushed her. We applied her makeup, instructing her each step of the way on what to do. We bought her a new hat, put some new big earrings in her ears and "Voilà!"—a new lease on life and on her situation. She was smiling from ear to ear and we were all laughing together again. Her mood had done a complete 180.

Fresh and Renewed

That is why I feel that this book is so important for me to write. I know that many of you do not have the great fortune of having a sister who is a hairdresser or a makeup artist. And I never want *any* woman to receive a look of pity because of the new appearance cancer has given her. This chapter will help you look fresh and renewed even when you do not feel that way.

So let's get busy!

WiseGeek.com states that one of the top reasons women wear makeup is "to enhance their natural beauty and be more physically alluring." Some women wear makeup because it gives us confidence. This does not mean we as women could not be confident without makeup. It simply serves as a boost for your natural self-confidence. (par. 1, 2)

We all have a self-image—a picture in our head of what we look like; and if we get sick, our bodies change, our appearance changes, and so does our self-image—often taking quite a blow, as any woman battling cancer will tell you.

While there is no evidence to suggest that looking good will speed up a cancer patient's recovery, a growing body of research indicates that understanding and effectively dealing with the changes in appearance that occur during cancer treatment may help patients better cope with their disease.

Chemotherapy can damage your self-image. It can change the hue of your skin, taking a healthy complexion to pale or ash or yellow, or worse. And in these cases, your present makeup may be of no use to you. Choose your new makeup to counteract these effects.

Shelf Life of Your Makeup... Should It Stay or Should It Go?

I am asked this question all the time: "Does my makeup ever go bad?"

As a matter of fact, it does. It does not matter how much you have paid for your makeup, it has a shelf life and an expiration date. During this time especially, you want to take every precaution to stay bacteria-free.

Here is what I have discovered about the life of your opened cosmetics:

Product	Expiration
Mascara	3 months
Liquid or cream foundation	12 months
Concealer	12 to 18 months
Powder/Powder foundation	18 months
Blush or Bronzer	18 months
Cream Blush	12 to 18 months
Eye Shadow	18 months
Eyeliner	18 months
Liquid Eyeliner	6 months
Lipstick/Lip Gloss	18 months
Lip Liner	12 months
Nail Polish	12 months

As a general rule, if your cosmetic has an odor or changes texture or becomes sticky or oily, it is best to throw it away. If you use an expired cosmetic, the best-case scenario is that it will be clumpy and less effective. The *worst-case scenario* is that it can cause a skin irritation, an allergic reaction, or even an infection, which is something that you certainly do not need to contend with during a cancer battle!

Never use eye makeup if you have an eye infection. The bacteria can contaminate your product and spread the infection to everything it touches. And this goes for any other type of infection when the makeup application cannot be done with a cotton ball, swab, or makeup sponge (i.e., lipstick, lip pencil, *eye* liner, mascara, etc.).

In addition, never share your makeup with others. The problems and chances of contamination here are numerous.

Things to Think about

1. **Use disposable applicators when applying your makeup.**
   Stocking up on cotton swabs and cotton balls is a good idea during this time. I know that this may seem like overkill, but your immune system can be very low right now. Remember that, in order to kill the bad cancer cells, some of your good cells have to be destroyed as well. Each time a makeup applicator touches your skin and then touches your eye shadow dispenser, let's say, any bacteria that was on your eyelid is now on your *eye* shadow and in its container. Now once or twice may not seem like much, but bacteria like to multiply; and if you do this day in and day out, you add additional bacteria each time. If you use a clean cotton swab each time you touch the *eye* shadow container, you are less likely to contaminate the product.
2. **Do not use your fingers to dispense product.**
   Let's say that your moisturizer is in a jar and you stick your finger in the jar to retrieve the product. Any bacteria or germs that are on your finger are now in the jar. Again, if you do this day after day, that is a lot of bacteria. Use a small makeup spatula to dispense a small amount of product. Use a clean spatula each time you use the cream or sanitize the spatula \with an alcohol swab.

3. **Sanitize your makeup brushes.**
   Alcohol is the cheapest and easiest way to sanitize your makeup brushes. Place two ounces of isopropyl alcohol in a spray bottle. Hold the bottle six to eight inches away from the brush head and spray two to three times. Then gently wipe the brush on a paper towel. This can be done daily to sanitize your brushes. Your makeup brushes should also be cleaned one to two times each month. This can be done with warm water and a facial cleanser. Remove the excess water and lay the brush flat to dry.

4. **Wash your hands.**
   Start by washing your hands with soap or antibacterial wash before applying your makeup. Now, on to the fun stuff… Let's play!

Steps for Your Makeup Application

Cleanse   Always use upward, circular movements.

Tone   Use a no-alcohol or very low-alcohol toner. Mist it onto your face or apply with a cotton ball.

Moisturize Dot the product on your forehead, cheeks, and chin to evenly distribute, and always use an upward, circular movement to work it into your skin.

Concealer   Use concealer on problem areas to blend the complexion evenly.

Foundation (sponge) Apply dots to your forehead, cheeks, and chin. Blend evenly. Pay close attention to the blend of the jaw line.

Powder   Apply with a brush that can be sanitized or with a cotton ball. Lightly dust entire face.

Blush	Apply with a brush that can be sanitized or with a cotton ball. Smile and apply blush from apple of the cheek to the hairline in an upward, circular motion. Blush not only adds color, but it also contours and defines your cheekbones. This can be very helpful when steroids give you a moon face. (If the blush is a cream, apply it before the powder.)
Eye Shadow	Refer to pages 112-116. Apply eye shadow with a cotton swab.
Eyeliner	Apply to lower lid under lashes, from the outer corner to ¾ of the way to the inside of the eye. On the upper lid, apply eyeliner at the lash line from corner to corner. This will give the illusion of eyelashes if there are none there.
Eyebrows	Apply to brow line using light, soft feathery strokes. (Refer to Eyebrows, pages 115.)
Mascara	If lashes are present, apply mascara to upper and lower lash line. When removing the mascara brush from tube to apply mascara, slowly turn the brush inside the tube as you remove it. Never push the brush rapidly in and out of the tube to apply more product to the brush. This action forces old mascara and bacteria deep into the tube.
Lip Liner	Draw a "V" along the top edge of Cupid's Bow. From the top corner of the "V," follow the line of the Vermillion Border to the corner of the mouth. Repeat for the opposite side. Draw a line from one corner of the lower lip, across the Lower Vermillion Border, to the middle of the lower lip on each side. Then fill the lip in with the liner.

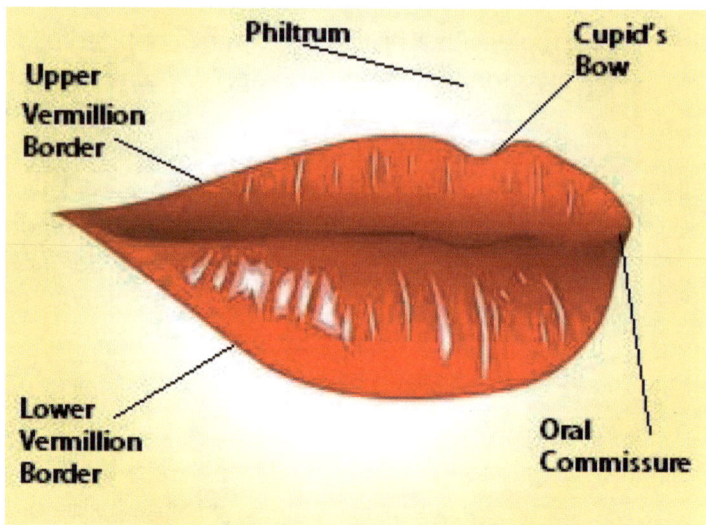

| Lip Stick | Apply lipstick over the top of the lip liner. |

Blush
- When applying blush, you want the color to look soft and natural, as if it comes from within.
- Tap or lightly blow on the applicator brush to remove any excess powder before applying, to prevent harsh and uneven application.
- Apply your blush on the apple of your cheek (the "apple" of your cheek pops out when you are smiling!) and, using an upward, circular motion, carefully blend toward your natural hairline.
- If two shades are being used, apply the darker one on the apple of your cheek first and then use the lighter shade to highlight. Blend well so there is no visible line between the colors.
- Highlight your temples, forehead, and chin with a light stroke of your blush brush or cotton ball.

Make sure to blend the blush into your foundation well or it will tend to look unnatural and add the appearance of five years to your looks.

How Do I Choose the Correct Cheek Color?

According to TheBeautyDepartment.com, certain shades of blush look better on your skin tone than others. You want your color to be more like a natural flush, as if you were blushing (thus, the name). Here are their suggestions for "The Most Harmonious Blush Shades for your Skin":

Skin Color	Blush Color
Porcelain	Apricot

Fair skin with warm undertones looks Gorgeous! with this peachy-yellow shade.

Ivory	Pale Pink

Fair skin with cool undertones naturally looks best with cool pink.

Beige	Amber

Medium skin tones with yellow or olive undertones look beautiful with these amber shades.

Tawny	Rose

Medium to dark skin tones with cool undertones work very well with the cool undertones of a rose cream blush.

Almond	Fuchsia

Dark skin tones with warm undertones surprisingly radiate more with cool bright pink blush shades than with warm ones.

Ebony	Tangerine

This time, the dark skin tone has cool undertones. As often happens with opposites, it goes with the warm blush.

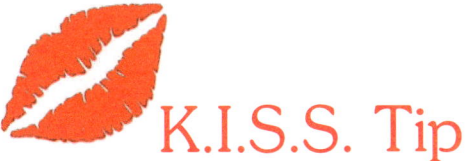

K.I.S.S. Tip

When you put on mascara, don't lower your chin—that's how mascara gets on your lid.

Eye Makeup

Here are a few hints and tips to personalize your makeup and make your eyes stand out. First, let's look at the different types of eyes:

Types of Eyes

Deep-Set Eyes

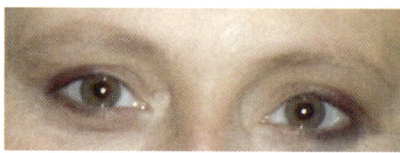

Deep-set eyes are large and set deeper into the skull, creating the illusion of a more prominent brow line. Dust medium shadow on the upper lid and crease. Add contour shade on the outer $1/3$ of the crease and add highlight just under the brow. Line the outer $1/2$ of the upper lid and extend slightly upward and soften the line.

Close-Set Eyes

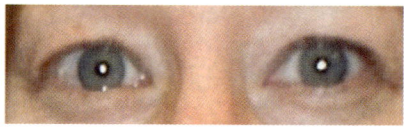

Close-set eyes are less than one eye length apart. Dust medium shadow over the lid. Apply a dark shade to the outer $1/3$ of the crease and blend outward at the outer edge of the eye. Add a highlight shadow to the brow bone at the eye's outer edge. Start $1/2$ way across with a liner and extend the liner just past the outer corner of the eye.

Wide-Set Eyes

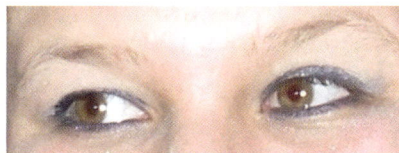

Wide-set eyes are more than one eye length apart. To bring them closer together, rim your top and bottom lash line with a black liner. Dust medium tone shadow over the entire lid. Apply dark shade in the crease from midway inward. Blend the hollow area from the nose to the brow. Highlight the brow bone at the brow arch.

Hooded Eyes

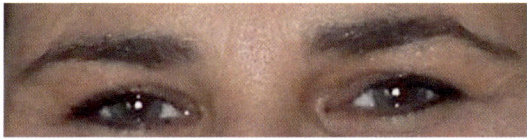

Hooded eyes feature an extra layer of skin that settles over the crease, causing the lid to appear smaller. To draw the focus upward, diffuse the darker shadow over and out past the crease. Dust the medium shadow from lash line to brow bone. Blend and fade toward the brow. Thicken the lashes at the base and draw a tight line across the top lash line to make your eyes appear larger. Curl lashes before applying mascara.

Downturned Eyes

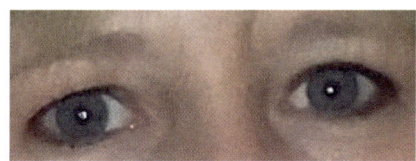

Downturned eyes drop slightly on the outer corners. To create that sexy cat's-eye look, apply a medium shade only from the inner edge of the iris to the bridge of the nose, then apply a liquid liner along the top lid until you get to the outer corner of the eye and finish with a small outward and upward flourish at a 45-degree angle.

Upturned Eyes

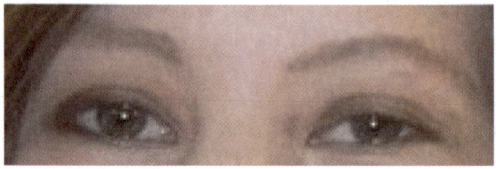

The upturned eye takes the form of a classic almond shape, with a natural lift at the outer corner. The lower lid looks longer than the top. Apply a dark shadow or pencil along the length of the outer, lower corner. Make sure you duplicate the effects on the upper lid by swiping the same eye shadow across the bottom lash line.

Mature Eyes

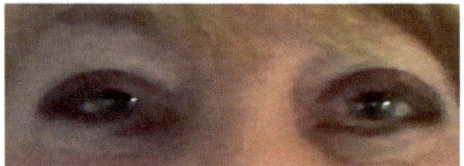

Mature eyes are the result of a loss of elasticity in your eyelids. Dust medium shade over the entire lid. Avoid dark shades in the crease and do not use highlighter unless the skin under the brow is taut. Use an eyeliner at the lash line and make the line thicker toward the outer ½ of the eye. Apply any color eyeliner at the lash line. Blend the line well into the shadow. Emphasize the upper lashes with mascara. Apply little or no mascara to the lower lashes. Do not put color over wrinkles, as it calls attention to them.

Also, remember these simple rules when applying eye makeup:
- When using colors, stick to sweeping one shade over the eye rather than several.
- Try using a dark tone as an eyeliner to emphasize the upper lash line by using the thin edge of a

disposable applicator to draw a soft line just above the upper lash.
- When applying shadow, apply over most of the eye area first, usually in a medium shade.
- Keep the principles of light and dark in mind while applying color. Dark color recedes and light brings them forward.

The Most Flattering Makeup Color for Your Eyes

If I have heard it once, I have heard it a thousand times:

"I don't wear makeup."

My response is always, "Ok, but now you do not have to do your hair, so you can fill that time by doing your makeup!"

Many of the women who have gone through our program come back to us years later and tell us that the day of their makeover was a turning point in their cancer journey, and sometimes in their life. We made them feel girly again. Take the time to take care of you. Do the things that make you feel girly!

Here are some hints and tips according to makeupgeek.com, to the most flattering eye shadows for your particular eye color:

Brown Eyes

Because brown is a neutral color, almost any color will make this eye color pop. The trick is finding which colors look best with your skin color as well. Generally, teals and purples look best on brown eyes.

Blue Eyes

Here is a tip that will make your blue eyes really stand out—wear colors that are opposite on the color wheel. Those would be golds, oranges, coppers, and browns. Blues can help blue eyes pop if it is a darker blue, and used in moderation. Purples will also make a statement.

Green Eyes

Stylemotivation.com states: "Green eyes are beautiful and deserve to be enhanced.... (M)akeup that is red-based bring(s) out your gorgeous green eyes. Bronze, copper and gold looks absolutely fabulous with green eyes for evening. Brown or dark green eye shadow with flecks of gold are also terrific choices."

Hazel Eyes

TypeF.com says: Spice up your hazel eyes with shadows in shades of bright green, lime green and even gold. Violet, plum and purple shades will bring contrast to your eyes, drawing out the vivid green shades in your hazel eyes.

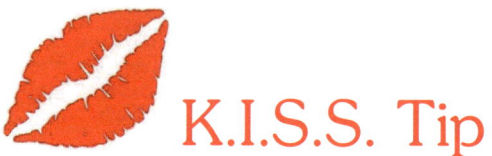

K.I.S.S. Tip

If you go bold and dramatic with your eyes, tone down the other areas of your makeup so that your eyes can POP!

Eyebrows

Have you ever thought to yourself, why do I have eyebrows? I think about silly stuff like that all the time. Eyebrows actually have a function. Eyebrows are on our face to prevent sweat, water or other debris from falling down into the eye socket. But, as we all have experienced, eyebrows are also very important to human communication and facial expression.

Eyebrows to me are one of the most important of makeup applications. I can pull my hair back off of my face and think to myself, "I would do okay without hair." But then I imagine myself without eyebrows and that is when I feel that I would look sick, that there is something wrong with me. This section will instruct how to draw a very natural looking eyebrow on and make it look proportional to your face. You will be surprised at how your sculpted eyebrow will add shape and color to your face.

Have your eyebrows thinned out, or fallen out completely? We can fix that, so let's get drawing!

Eyebrows that may not be there can be created by using the four-point system. The use of an eyeliner or eyebrow pencil and the tip of the nose as your stationary point can create a realistic-looking eyebrow.

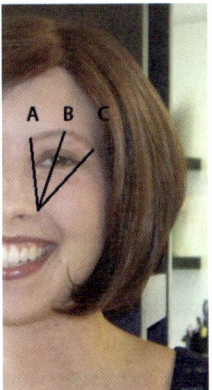

1. Take the liner straight up from side of the nose and make a dot, at the brow bone. Call this point "A."
2. Holding the liner at the side of the nose, slide the opposite end of the liner across the center of the eye and make a dot (Arch of the Eyebrow). Call this point "B."
3. Holding the liner at the side of the nose, slide across the corner of the eye at the end of the brow bone and make a dot. Call this point "C."
4. Now, using the eyeliner or brow pencil and a very light, feathery stroke, "connect the dots"; A to B, B to C, then give the drawn eyebrow some natural width and shape using that same light and feathery stroke. This will create a very soft and natural-looking eyebrow.

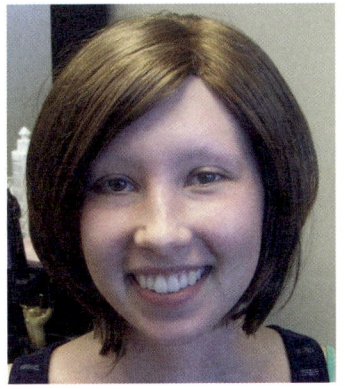

Melissa Before

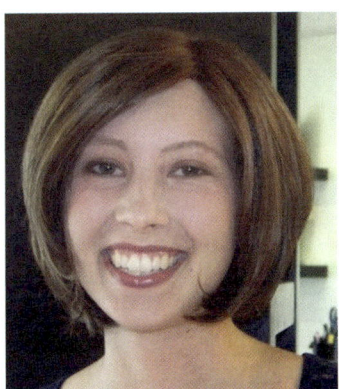

Melissa After

Eyebrow Stencils

These are plastic stencils that resemble the shape of your eyebrow. They range from thin to thick. The stencil is held over the existing eyebrow, and then a powder is brushed over the stencil to give a new, more perfect shape to your eyebrows.

I love products like this. There is only one problem for the special people going through treatment: there need to be eyebrows for the powder to stick to. Once they begin to grow back, this is a great way to add some definition to a thin brow. But drawing your eyebrows on freehand is still the best way to create real-looking eyebrows on someone without them.

False Eyelashes

I feel that false eyelashes are too risky while going through chemotherapy and radiation.

1. You may have a reaction to the adhesive.
2. You may have a reaction to the adhesive remover.
3. If the eyelashes are removed improperly, an open wound may occur and that could be a source of infection.

I understand that there will be special occasions for which you want to look your best—and I am all for the exceptions—but, as a rule, I would advise you to stay away from false eyelashes until your treatment has been completed.

Mascara

Mascara is a cosmetic commonly used to enhance the eyes by darkening, thickening, lengthening and/or defining the eyelashes.

According to Squidoo.com, there are 5 different types of mascara. What you need to decide is what you want your lashes to do, and then you can choose a mascara by its merits. Choosing is now much more of a challenge because there are so many types from which to choose.

The 5 Types of Mascara:

Lengthening Mascara

This type has a brush with longer bristles. These help to deposit more mascara on the tips of your lashes for the purpose of extending the length of the eyelashes.

Thickening Mascara

Thickening mascara wands are made with thick bristles. They also contain a mixture of silicone or other types of waxes which help to gain a thicker form. If you were looking to broaden your eyelashes and make them stand out more by thickening them, this is the product for you.

Waterproof Mascara

Waterproof mascara is excellent if you do not want to ruin your mascara effect out in the rain or water. However, these types of mascaras can cause your lashes to break off. It needs to be removed with an eye makeup remover.

Curling Mascara

When curling your eyelashes, you curl them up and away, thereby exposing your eyes to give them better definition and adding thickness to the lashes at the same time.

Defining Mascara

Defining mascara coats each lash to make them dramatically long, extremely defined and visually separated. (par. 4)

Lipstick

Why do women feel better when they wear lipstick? It definitely adds color to a sometimes not-so-colorful face. Lipstick symbolizes sex appeal and draws attention to one of the most sensual features of a woman. The traditional reason women wore lipstick was to disguise sexual stimulation. When women get excited their lips turn redder, due to increased blood flow. So, in a more reserved age, this coloring was added to hide the inadvertent reddening of the lips and, over the years, this has evolved into a fashion statement. Makeup, in general, is seen to enhance the beauty of a woman. Lipstick enhances the shape and color of a woman's lips.

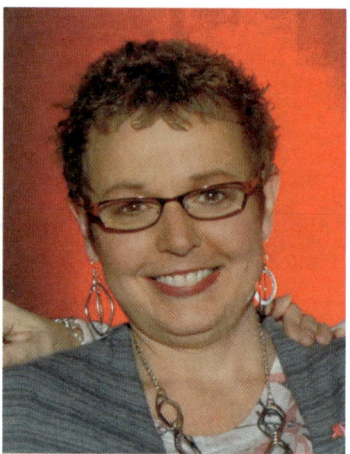

Lynne's lipstick is Gorgeous!

The Correct Shade of Lipstick for You

According to makeup artist Bobbi Brown, the most flattering lipstick tones for you will be one or two shades darker than your natural lip color. To test shades, apply the lipstick or lip gloss to one lip and compare it to the other. If it appears one to two shades darker than your natural color, you have a winner!

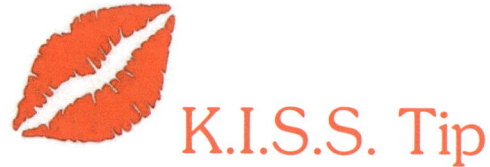

K.I.S.S. Tip

Wearing blush and lipstick can make you look younger—even if that is the only makeup you wear!

"The question isn't who's going to let me; it's who is going to stop me."

– Ayn Rand

Chapter 11

Let's Play Dress-Up!

Time to talk fashion! We touch on different body shapes, what is best for your body type, what colors look best on you, and that you should stick to what you are comfortable with but also be open to new things.

Make fashion your friend and do not overthink it. Remember...

Go! Set! Ready!

*"**Dress shabbily and they remember the dress. Dress impeccably, and they remember the woman.**"*
– Coco Chanel

Fashion

For eons, societies and their citizens have used clothes and other body decoration not only as modest coverings and protection from the elements, but also as a form of nonverbal communication. Fashion can indicate occupation, rank, availability, locality, class, wealth, and gender. Those with high status occupations will wear the clothes they think others expect them to wear. And it is from a person's clothing that we can get our first impression of their personality.

Do you remember when we were five-year-old little girls and played "Dress-Up"? I remember getting into my mom's closet and pulling one of her dresses off of the hanger and stepping into it. Next, it was finding a pair of her high heels that I would then clomp to the bathroom in, to find her lipstick—to put all the way around my lips just to make sure that my lips were good and covered. I loved to play dress-up. I used to think that I was a princess. I am sure I did not look like a princess, with clothes that were way too big and lipstick all over my face, but I did *feel* like one. I believe that *that* is why fashion is so important in today's world.

Fashion is a general term for a popular style or practice, especially in clothing, shoes, makeup, and accessories. Fashion is defined as a distinctive and often habitual trend in style in which a person dresses.

Why is fashion so important? According to Wikipedia.com, fashion is ultimately important because it is a form of communication. You are communicating to others who are important to you. Around the start of the 20th century, fashion style magazines began to include pictures and became even more influential. In cities throughout the world these magazines were greatly sought after and had a profound effect on people's taste.

In the 1920s, Coco Chanel was a major figure in fashion—at the time as much for her magnetic personality as for her chic and progressive designs. Chanel helped to popularize the bob hairstyle, the little black dress, and the use of jersey knit for women's clothing.

According to Ask.com, clothing does more than just conceal your body. It has the ability to accentuate your figure and to minimize your flaws. It can give you a carefree image, one of professionalism, or anything in between—whatever suits your lifestyle. Your fashion can make you feel your best and boost your confidence. It sets the tone for who you are.

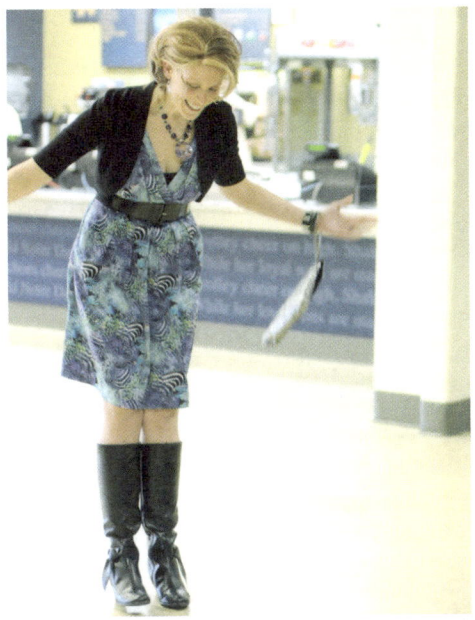

Kendelle

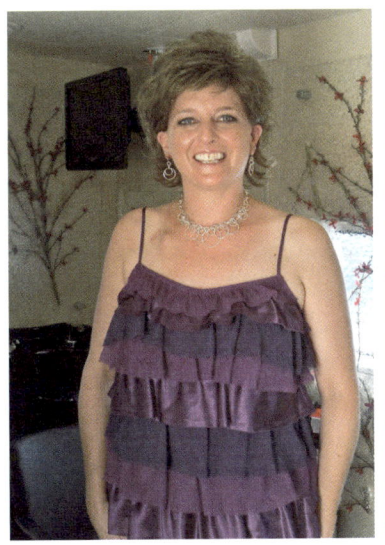

Elise

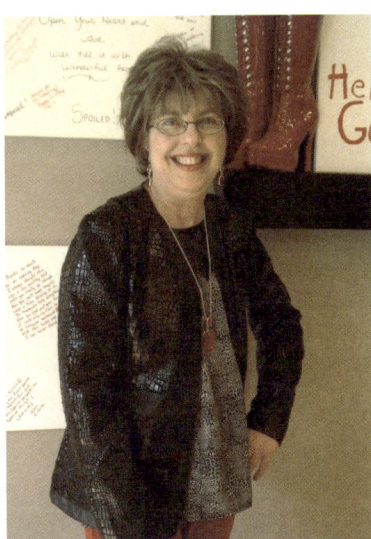

Anne

Kristi's Story

For the past few years we have performed a makeover at the "Pink Zone Game," a women's collegiate basketball game played at the University of Notre Dame to support the fight against breast cancer. We pre-arrange to surprise a breast cancer survivor in the audience prior to the start of the game and give her a surprise makeover while the basketball game is going on, with her reveal done on center court in front of 10,000 people before the end of the game. It is a makeover on overdrive and it is an awesome experience for the recipient. She receives a manicure, pedicure, facial, a new outfit, a wig if she needs one, and her makeup is done.

While planning the makeover during the months before the game, I have many conversations with the individual who nominated the woman battling cancer. One of the questions that we ask, among others, is about her clothing sizes and style. We want to make sure that she feels like a million dollars after her makeover, so she has to feel confident with our clothing choices for her.

When the subject of clothing style was discussed for the Pink Zone Game recipient this year, we were told that Kristi was "a sweatshirt and jeans kind of gal." In other words, she was a very casual dresser. Kristi was a teacher by profession, used to being in the public eye, so I had a feeling that she liked dressing up when she had the opportunity. We decided to pick out three outfits that were casual but dressier than her nominator was suggesting. After the facial, manicure, and pedicure, we have our Gorgeous Woman model the outfits that we have chosen for her. And as Kristi tried on the dressier outfits we had chosen, it was as if a light went on inside of her! Kristi pranced around the room, over and over, and her smile was contagious. She would walk up to her family and say, "Feel my butt in these jeans!!!" It was an incredible transformation to watch. I was glad I followed my instincts and gave her the opportunity to dress up.

Kristi told us how good it felt to get dressed up. She told us that during your cancer battle, you just do not always feel like putting on nice clothes. She had forgotten how good it felt. Kristi felt so good that she danced in Center Court during her Reveal that day, in front of a sold-out crowd.

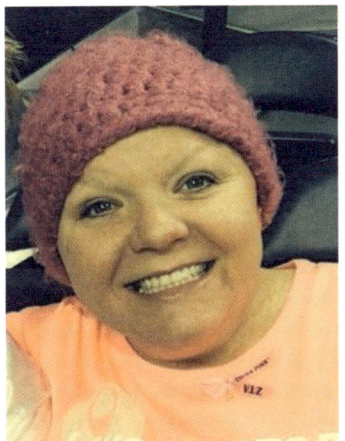
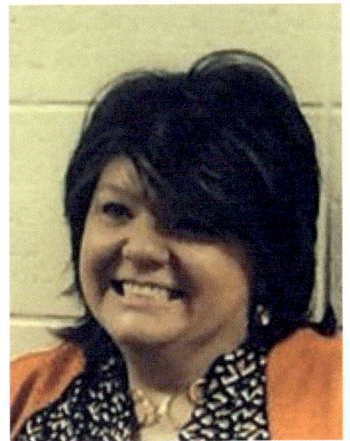

Kristi Before   Kristi After

Don't Wait for the Perfect Moment

So let's talk about clothes. Years ago I went to a presentation by Winn Claybaugh—author, motivational speaker, and founder and co-owner of hair care giant Paul Mitchell's beauty school division, with more than 100 locations throughout the United States. Many of us in the room were young hairdressers, just starting out in our careers. He began to talk about how it was our job as a hairdresser to make people look good, which made them feel good about themselves. However, unless we felt good about *ourselves*, there was no way that we could do our job effectively. I remember to this day Winn saying: "Everything in your closet should make you feel like a million dollars! Am I telling you to get rid of everything that doesn't make you feel that way and buy all new clothes? YES I AM!"

I was young and thought to myself, "This guy is nuts! I cannot spend $1,000 on myself for new clothes." I could not wrap my brain around it. Then my thoughts went in another direction, "Why *can't* I spend money for new clothes? Why do I not deserve a new wardrobe? How better would I serve my clients if I felt good about myself every day?"

Let me share something with you. I love Chico's, the clothing store. I love their style of clothing. It looks very classy to me and not too stuffy. My goal was to have a closet filled with nothing but clothes from Chico's. I have treated myself to one new outfit every year for the last seven years. I shop at the Chico's outlet stores to add to my existing collection once or twice a year as well. One day I happened to pay attention to what was hanging in my closet. Seventy percent of what was in my closet was all from Chico's. I could not believe it. However, I purposely wore the Chico's clothes only on special occasions or for speaking engagements. WHAT!?!?! WAKE UP, KIM!!!!

Kristi taught me a great lesson that day of her visit, and it reminded me of an anonymous quote I had heard years before:

"Do not wait for the perfect moment.
Take the moment and make it perfect."

Every day is special. Here it was, I had an entire closet filled with clothes that made me feel classy and vivacious and yet I never wore them except for speaking engagements and special events.

Treat every day as a gift. Do something today and every day that makes you feel like a million dollars. Wear high heels with your jeans. Break out that special colorful shirt that you wear only to weddings. Start wearing those diamond earrings that you wear only on your anniversary and put on some RED LIPSTICK!!

Body Image

I feel very strongly about including a section on fashion and the different body types. For many women, during cancer their body type remains practically unchanged. But there are some women whose body type will change due to weight gain, weight loss, or surgery.

This became very apparent to me at one of our surprise makeovers. We orchestrated it at one of our affiliate salons. Mandy was a breast cancer survivor who was just a little thing, but God had blessed Mandy with a very large chest. Her pant size was a 2, but her shirt size was an extra-large. Because of her cancer diagnosis, it was recommended that Mandy have a mastectomy on the breast affected with cancer and a reduction in the other breast. As I stated, Mandy wore a size 2 in pants, but she carried some extra weight right around her middle. However, due to the size of her breasts she never took notice of that extra weight. All of a sudden her body shape—and the image she had of her body—completely changed.

After surgery, Mandy's chest was much smaller, which made her midsection appear much more prominent, and it made her self-conscious. So we chose an outfit for Mandy that she was comfortable in, but positively accentuated her new figure. We chose a pair of jeans that showed off her slim hips and a longer shirt with three-quarter-length sleeves that hit right at her hips. Then we added a longer necklace, matching bracelets and big earrings to pull the entire look together. Mandy was so happy that she could not stop smiling.

Knowing your body type, and how to dress for it, is a strength we all need. This section will give all of you some tips in that area.

> *Trisha Greenlee*, Creative Director for Hello Gorgeous!, suggests that layering your clothes is a good idea while you are going through treatment.
>
> "Your body temperature can fluctuate quickly from hot to cold, so many thin layers will allow you to more easily regulate your temperature by removing a little or a lot."
>
> She continues by saying, "It is very easy to layer your clothing. Start with a tank top, add a long-sleeved blouse, buttoned half-way up, and place a sweater over that." She also included that buttoning just a few buttons in the middle of your blouse or your jacket will show off your waist. And utilize your accessories such as earrings, bracelets and scarves to enhance your current look.

Fashion and Body Shapes

Have you ever experienced how a certain jacket looks great on one of your girlfriends, so you search to find the exact jacket in the exact color—only to find that it looks hideous on you? It can work the other way as well.

Before delving into a style journey it is important to know, and understand what looks good on, your body. This implies knowing your body and what pieces can enhance or hide certain areas. This section will help you best define your body type, which will enable you to accentuate the positives and downplay the negatives.

God created us all differently, which is one reason why women come in all different shapes and sizes. Every fashion website, book, magazine, and blog seems to have a slightly different idea about the best way to describe these different female body types. And so, influenced by more than a dozen different websites and book sources, here are brief descriptions for each body type—and suggestions on how to flatter each one.

Finding Your Body Type

Once you know your body type, it will be much easier to find clothes that flatter you. Here is a simple way to determine the shape of your body.

First, take a measurement of your bust, waist, and hips, and write the measurements down. Then read the section below to determine the body type that best describes your shape. I have chosen the five primary body types—each one based on the main area your body tends to store its fat deposits. The five main body types are: Rectangle, Pear, Hourglass, Apple and Strawberry.

Rectangle Body Shape

✦ Your waist will measure up to nine inches smaller than your hips or bust.

Rectangle

The Rectangle body shape (also known as the Straight body type) visually displays proportion between your shoulders and hips, both of which can be full-figured or flat. This body type can make you look shorter and heavier than you actually are. Over 45% of American women have a rectangle body type. This means that your hips and bust are balanced and your waist is not very defined. You tend to gain weight in your torso first, and your arms and legs are typically slender. Your lower legs are shapely and your best feature.

How to Dress the Rectangle Body Shape

The key to dressing a Rectangle body type is to proportionately dress the top and the bottom of your body in a way that will enhance your waist. To create a more curvaceous effect, add volume (or the illusion of volume) proportionately to the upper and lower body by mixing and matching separates.

Tops

Look for tops that will add curves to your upper half and create a more defined waist. A great addition is a top with a belt or one that has a wide V- or U-neck.

Bottoms

Look for bottoms that add curves to your lower half while creating an hourglass shape. Look for full-flared legs and high- or low-rise waistbands.

Rectangle Body Shapes Should Avoid:
- Figure-hugging garments
- Drop waistlines
- Bulky, heavy textures
- Double-breasted jackets

Pear Body Shape

✦ Your hips are larger than your bust and your waist is nicely defined.

Pear

The Pear body shape, also known as the Triangle, is defined by a fuller butt, hips, and thighs; a narrower bust to hips ratio with a defined waistline. You have an elegant neck and proportionately slim arms and shoulders. You first gain weight in your legs and rear end and your waist is your best asset.

How to Dress the Pear Body Shape

The key to dressing a pear-shape is to enhance and add volume to the upper body, while emphasizing your waist and deemphasizing your lower body to create a balanced, hourglass appearance.

Tops

Look for tops that will help balance your lower half while accentuating your defined waist. Look for bright colors and bold patterns.

Bottoms

Look for bottoms that will minimize your lower half such as A-line skirts. Stick with darker colors, clean lines, and simple stitching.

Pear Body Shapes Should Avoid:

- Cropped pants
- Wide flared legs
- Kitten heels
- Mini-skirts
- Pencil skirts

Hourglass Body Shape

✦ Your hips and bust are almost equal in size with a narrow waist.

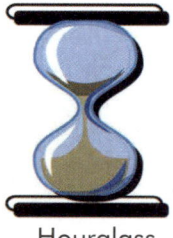

Hourglass

The Hourglass is the ideal figure. It is associated with a perfectly proportionate bust line and hips and a well-defined waist. Fat deposits evenly above and below your waist. You have the hourglass shape that most women dream of. Your bust and hips are well-balanced and you have a beautifully defined waist. Your upper body is proportionate in length to your legs, which are shapely. You are in balance from top to bottom.

How to Dress the Hourglass Body Shape

The key to dressing for this shape is to proportionately dress the top and the bottom body while accentuating your waist.

Tops

Look for tops that will accentuate your waist and maintain the balanced look of your figure. Look for wrap-around styles, tailored jackets and shirts.

Bottoms

Lucky You!!! You can wear most any bottoms as long as you pair them with the right top. Try skinny jeans and skirts that show off your legs.

Hourglass Body Shapes Should Avoid:
- Any style or garment that hides your body shape

Apple Body Shape

✦ Your waist measurement is greater than your hips or your bust.

If you have the Apple body shape, your waist is undefined and you carry most of your weight around your midsection. This body shape is sometimes divided into two types, Diamond and

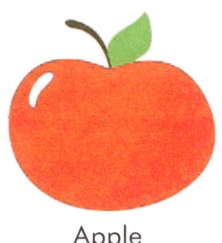

Apple

Oval—the diamond body shape being defined by a high stomach, while the oval body type means you carry your weight low. Most Apple body shapes have a full bust and great legs.

How to Dress the Apple Body Shape

The key to this body shape is to de-emphasize your midsection and create a more defined waist.

Tops

Look for tops that will taper your upper body while creating a more defined waist. Look for vertical details or patterns. Tops that flare at the hips and have a square, wide U-, or V-neckline will look great.

Bottoms

Look for bottoms that will minimize your lower half but will balance the upper body with the lower body. Wide-waistband and wide, full-leg pants will create balance as well as flared or bubble skirts.

Apple Body Shapes Should Avoid:
- Skirts above the knee
- Sleeves that finish next to the bust
- Double-breasted coats or jackets
- High-waisted pants
- Excessive fabric at the midsection

Strawberry Body Shape

✦ You have large shoulders and/or bust with narrow hips.

The Strawberry or Inverted Triangle is the exact opposite of the Pear. Some consider this body type to be the most ideal—a full bust line with a defined waist and narrow hips. This build is characterized by broad shoulders and is often associated with

Strawberry

athletes. These are the girls we refer to as "top heavy." To balance this out, try bright-colored or patterned fabrics. Full skirts will add more body below the waist.

How to Dress the Strawberry Body Shape

The key to dressing this shape is the balance of your shoulders and bust with your hips, while creating a waist. Choose clothing that adds curves and fullness to the lower body.

Tops

Find tops that will create a more defined waist and accentuate your shoulder and bust. Wide V-necks and U-necks work well.

Bottoms

Fuller skirts and wide-leg trousers will help you balance your body shape beautifully.

Strawberry Body Shapes Should Avoid:

- Shoulder pads
- Tapering trousers
- Puffy sleeves
- Halter necks
- Pencil skirts
- Skinny jeans

Leeca – Manager, Maurice's

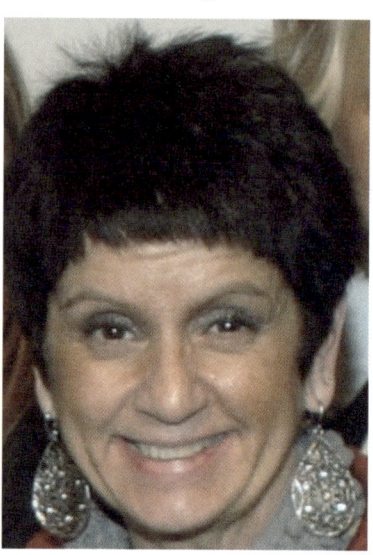

(Leeca, from Maurice's, is the very first manager we approached to help us with the outfit for a Gorgeous! Woman Makeover, during our 6-week Tour in 2010. And, as it is with many things in life—the first is the best! Leeca has a passion for these women on the same level as our Affiliate Salon owners. She is priceless!)

I am so grateful for all of my experiences with Hello Gorgeous! I have been given the chance to help change a life for one day of women who are in the battle of their lives. And for a few hours on that one day, we make their lives better, we give them a more beautiful outlook, and hopefully they see themselves in a different light. I was very lucky to get to do so many Reveals for so many special women.

I think one of the best things that has happened is that I met Kim and Mike and Trisha—I feel like family with them and I have become a better person by knowing them. Now I look at people in need and I see opportunities of how I can help them that I hadn't seen before. Every story and memory I have of the Reveals bring tears, but they are all good tears, and they are just a sign of how much passion goes into each Reveal. I love you guys and please keep me at the top of your list when you need my help.

— Leeca Smith

As you can see, there are advantages to every body shape and techniques for each woman to use fashion to accentuate the good traits and conceal the weaknesses. You will be surprised what these small changes can do for your image, your figure and your confidence!

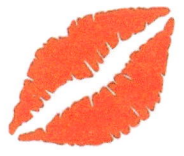 K.I.S.S. Tip

"Always organize your clothes going light to dark from left to right in your closet. Your eye will follow the color and thus help you stay organized."

— Melanie Charlton Fascitelli
Founder, Clos-ette and Clos-ette Too

"As a woman, I believe you have to embrace your body, and feel beautiful both inside and out."

— Tamara Ecclestone

Chapter 12

Showing One's True Colors

Matching the right clothing colors to your skin tone is something that women depend on to look their best. Most of you know instinctively what colors you look best in; but cancer treatment can change your base skin tone during this time, which sometimes leaves your favorite colors out in the cold.

This section gives you the fashion guru's guide to what colors go with each skin tone, and hints and tips to keep you looking Gorgeous, even if your skin tone changes for a while.

> *"A dress is a piece of ephemeral architecture, designed to enhance the proportions of the female body."*
>
> – Christian Dior

What's the Best Color for You?

All skin tones are either "warm" or "cool." Warmer tones are more yellow while cool skin has a pink or blue tone.

While going through your cancer treatment there is no reason why you cannot still look your best. You may not *feel* your best, but we can help make you look like a million bucks. By choosing the best clothing colors for your particular skin tone, you will:

- Make your skin glow;
- Make your eyes sparkle and shine;
- Make yourself look years younger;
- Gain compliments on how good you look, giving you added confidence;
- Make your entire appearance look complete.

By choosing the wrong colors for your skin tone, it can:
- Dull your complexion;
- Make you appear tired;
- Make you look older than you actually are;
- Give the illusion of added weight (which no one wants).

What Is My Proper Skin Tone?

Your underlying skin tone plays a huge part in determining what colors will look best on you. To test your underlying skin color:

- Pinch the skin on your ear lobe, the back of your hand, or the tip of your finger for a count of five.
- The skin color you see there for the following few seconds is your underlying skin tone.

If you see blue, pink, red, violet, or rosy tones, you will look best in cool colors. If you see peach, golden, warm red, or a coral tone, warm colors will be the best choice for you.

Jewelry Test

If you look good in silver jewelry, you more than likely have a cool undertone. If you look better in gold, your undertone is most likely warm.

The Compliment Test

One of the best ways to know that you are on the right track with the color of clothing you have chosen is to pay attention to the compliments you receive and what you are wearing when you receive them. For example, I once had a beautiful royal blue pantsuit. When I wore that suit, I received compliments on the color of my hair, the color of my eyes, and my skin tone. I always received numerous compliments each time I wore that suit. To me, that confirmed that my skin tone had a cool undertone and therefore I would seek out other pieces of clothing that had that color palette in them.

Here are some examples of warm and cool tones:

Warm Tones
Yellow
Orange
Brown
Yellow/Green
Orange/ Red

Cool Tones
Blue
Green
Pink
Purple
Magenta
Blue/Green
Blue/Red

Here are some other examples of the correct color for common skin tones and hair colors. Remember that all of these are *general guidelines*. Experiment yourself to find your perfect colors:

Olive skin tones look beautiful in pastels, light yellow, baby blue, mint green and light pink.

Gray-Haired Girls should wear dark-rimmed glasses to add color to their face and contrast with the lack of pigment in their hair. Dark shades like navy, black, chocolate brown, deep rose, and plum really set off a classic look on someone with gray hair. These ladies should also stay away from pastels.

Women with light hair and light eyes will look best in pastels and neutral colors. Strong colors like orange should be avoided.

Redheads are considered warm, especially if their eyes are brown and their skin has freckles. Emerald green and cobalt blue are stunning colors on redheads. These skin tones should avoid dull colors, browns and oranges.

The Seasons Are the Key

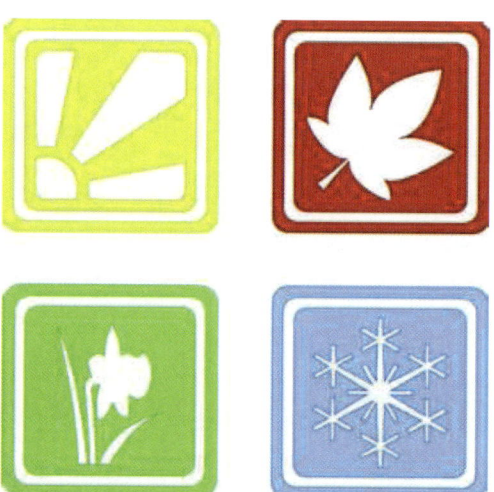

John Barrymore, writer for the website HowStuffWorks.com, writes, "We all have certain colors that we like to wear more than others. Interestingly, there's a reason for that. Depending on the color of our skin, certain colors can make us look pale or tan. They can help hide our flaws or make them more noticeable." (par. 1)

Mr. Barrymore goes on to say: "All skin types can be boiled down to four categories. These categories happen to correspond with the four seasons: winter, summer, autumn and spring. By matching your skin tone with the right season, you'll be able to dress your best." (par. 2)

In general, light skin tones look best with dark colors, medium skin tones look best with the primary colors and darker skin tones look best with whites and pale colors. As I understand the concept:

Spring skin tones are lighter, with a hint of freckles. You should wear yellows, blues and greens. Black and white should be avoided.

Summer skin tones are pink, which means that pastels work best for you and you should stay away from orange and black.

Fall skin tones are usually comprised of redheads and brunettes. They look best in oranges, browns and other earth tones, but (like those with spring skin tones) they should stay away from black and white.

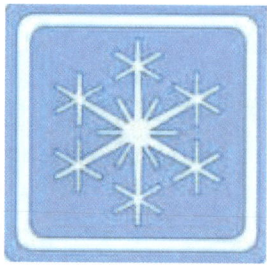

Winter skin tones can be pale, yellow, or dark with blue or pink undertones. Sharper colors like black and blue work well with this skin tone, but stay away from light browns.

I think that, if you are able to use these ideas as guidelines, you will be able to stay Gorgeous! through this transition. Most complexions and skin tones return to normal as your body slowly rids itself of the effects of your chemotherapy. So, for most of you, your favorite colors to wear will still be your favorites again.

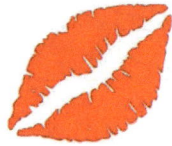

K.I.S.S. Tip

Buying neutral-colored shoes because they "go with everything" is safe but BORING. Pick something in a bold color and you will be surprised at how many outfits they will work with!

> *"I like light, color and luminosity. I like those things full of color and vibrance."*
>
> – Oscar de la Renta

Chapter 13

Celebrate!

We have covered a lot of material in the way of beauty. Now it is time to put it to the test. You can be transformed, just like our other Gorgeous! Women, and with a little extra work, you can gain some of that normalcy that you long to have back in your life.

We are empowering you with the knowledge. Now, let's get it done and celebrate your success!

> *"A woman whose smile is open and whose expression is glad has a kind of beauty no matter what she wears."*
>
> – Anne Roiphe

The Need to Celebrate!

When we first started Hello Gorgeous! we did things very differently. We did not have the mobile DaySpas. We would perform the visits in our salon. Our Gorgeous! Women received a special day of pampering, but with no outfit and no Reveal Party.

On one of our first year's visits, we surprised our Gorgeous! Woman while she was out for breakfast. We gave her our card and asked her to call us when she was ready for her makeover. She called and we planned a beautiful day for her—and we all had a great time. When we finished with our Gorgeous! Woman, though, we found out that, as good as she looked and felt, she had to go home to her ex-husband and her nine-year-old son. She would see no one who would truly appreciate her new look with her. So that day, when I got home, I told my husband Mike that there needed to be more to this day for these women. It just did not feel "finished." We decided that this special day of theirs needed to be *celebrated*.

Are you familiar with the old saying, "All dressed up and no place to go"? We needed to give these amazing women someplace to go—to show off their new look and to celebrate life with people who would share their enthusiasm. And I want to encourage you to celebrate *your* life as well. You are still here. You are winning. Find a way to celebrate your life every day.

Educating and Empowering Experience

"To create a unique *Experience* for women battling all types of cancers that *Empowers* these women through *Education* of cosmetic techniques and the use of products to bring back some of the femininity that cancer has taken from them."

This is the mission statement of the *Hello Gorgeous! Affiliate Salon Program*. The men and women who participate in our program do so voluntarily and their goal is to give you your POWER back and to celebrate it! We are speaking here about leverage.

Definition of Leverage (n)

1. power to get things done: power over other people, especially something that gives an advantage but is not referred to openly

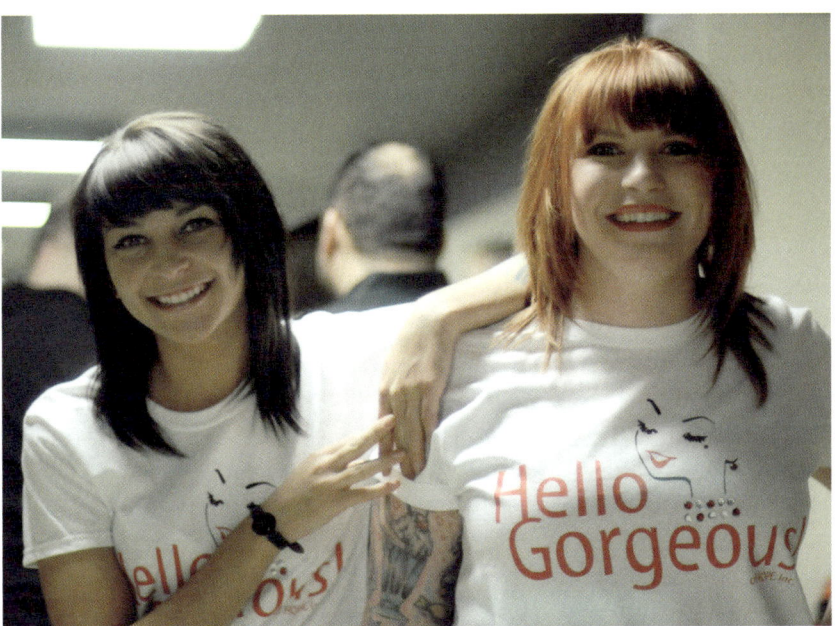

Cassie and Erica from FIX Salon/Spa

Leverage gives you an edge over a situation. It empowers you to succeed. All of the tips and procedures in this book are just that—leverage over the physical changes from your cancer treatment.

But the use of makeup, wigs, and fashion is only one part. The second part is the right attitude, positive thinking, and visualizing yourself *there*, wherever your there happens to be. The third part is to celebrate what you have now in your life. Celebrate it *every* day.

Do not get caught up in the *When-Then Cycle*. What is that, you ask?

When-Then Cycle

In the summer of 2013, I attended a seminar in Stamford, Connecticut, where I met many wonderful individuals. Two people, however, stuck out to me. Chris and Nancy are the owners of Income 180. These wonderful people are life coaches—they help you achieve what you want to achieve. And they have helped women entrepreneurs radically change their results in business. As we chatted, they explained to me the "When-Then" cycle and that

I was in the midst of this cycle, which I did not even know existed. They went on to explain that most people do not realize they are creating this cycle in themselves—this endless cycle that keeps them on the proverbial hamster wheel; round and round and never getting anywhere. For me, it was my public speaking career.

I always said that I wanted to lose 50 pounds before I would start to market myself as a public speaker; but, by waiting to lose the weight, I was just putting off my dream. I was waiting for the *when*, which I was nowhere near. So, *when* I lose 50 pounds, *then* I will start as a public speaker. As I stood there and listened, they suggested that I book my first speaking engagement *now*. Book it four months out from today, *but get it on the books*. Because, when it is on your calendar, then you have committed to it. So if weight loss was my goal, I needed to start right now because I now have a deadline. So many times, we wait for the *when*, which never comes, and it keeps us from the *THEN*!

Mark Batterson is the pastor of National Community Church in Washington, D.C., and one of my favorite authors. His books have touched my life exactly when I needed them. I had the opportunity to attend one of his services recently. I met him afterward to personally say thank you and told him how his writings have inspired me. The sermon that he gave the day that I met him spoke about this very thing. He explained that his church, NCC, has a little motto that has become a part of their mindset:

GO! SET! READY!

Mark further explains that, if we wait until we are ready, we will be waiting for the rest of our lives. He explains that in several places in the Bible, Jesus says, "GO." Jesus does not say, "Prepare, then go," He says "GO." Were you ready to get married? I thought that I had met my soul mate when I had met Mike, but I cannot say that I was *ready* to get married. And, like for most people, marriage was a challenge and it took a while for everything to run the way it was supposed to. But I am so glad that I ran past my fear of the unknown and married Mike. I can say that I was not ready to have a child, even being married for nine years prior to our son's birth. I did not feel that we had enough money in our savings account to support a child and care for him the way we wanted to. Then one day one of my clients said to me, "If you wait to have a baby until you think you are ready, you will never have a baby." Our son is the light of our lives and I cannot imagine our world without the endless banter that fills the back seat of our car and the joy of being a mom that fills my heart. The point is, if you wait for the perfect conditions to get married, have a baby, go on a vacation, or start a business, *it will never happen.*

I have watched someone battle a disease for 18 years with grace and style. I have watched my husband lie in a hospital bed with a fever of 104°, a catheter and an IV, while editing our first book on the computer and answering his cell phone with "Hello Gorgeous!" and a smile. Mike has a saying:

Walk the dog. Don't let the dog walk you.

Do not let your cancer diagnosis stall your dreams. Take as your example the amazing women in this book. Keep traveling, planting flowers, and filling your social calendar. Keep your standing appointment at your hair salon, if just to have your stylist shampoo your scalp and keep that salon socialization in your life. Keep dreaming and planning. Treat cancer as an inconvenience. And CELEBRATE! Celebrate your victories, celebrate every day. Find the joy in life and it will find you.

And for goodness sakes, make sure you wear your lipstick, ALL OF THE TIME! Not just when you go somewhere. Not when you arrive. Wear it *all* of the time. It is very empowering!!! Make a promise to wear your lipstick every day!!!

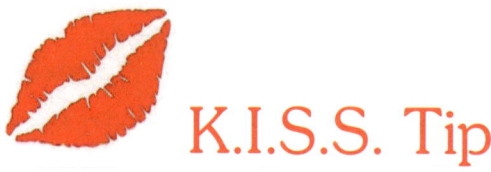 ## K.I.S.S. Tip

How to avoid getting lipstick on your teeth? After applying your lipstick, make a wide "O" letter with your lips, insert your clean first finger, close the "O" lightly around your finger and draw it outward, and then see the excess of lipstick stay on your finger (it would have eventually ended up on your teeth!).

> *"We delight in the beauty of the butterfly, but rarely admit the changes it has gone through to achieve that beauty."*
>
> – Maya Angelou

Chapter 14

Inspirational Stories

Over the course of the eight years that we have been doing Makeovers on these amazing Gorgeous! Women, we have always hoped that we would educate them on what they needed to know to appear Gorgeous anytime they wished; reconnect them with their family and friends through the Reveal Party experience; and empower them with the knowledge that these changes that they were experiencing could be overcome, and that they could persevere every day. We just never expected how much our three hours of service to each of these women would completely transform *us* forever—for the better—and inspire us to strive so hard to build this program.

So that *you* will understand just how important this work is to us, here are just a few of the inspiring stories we wish to share with you that have changed our lives so profoundly.

> *"When we love, we always strive to become better than we are. When we strive to become better than we are, everything around us becomes better too."*
>
> – Paulo Coelho

Kendelle
Cover Girl

My name is Kendelle Niespodziany and I am a wife, mother, daughter, sister, granddaughter, aunt, friend and so much more...and I am in treatment for breast cancer...again!

My journey began in 2012, at the age of 29, when I first heard those words no woman wants to hear, "You have breast cancer." I cried, yelled, and had all the normal reactions one would think you would have. Then at some point you have that moment where you just have to get in gear and do what is needed.

I had a lumpectomy, chemotherapy, double mastectomy, several of what I refer to as "tweaking surgeries" on my new girls (my implants), and physical therapy. Throughout all this I was privileged to meet so many special people who helped change my life forever. I survived and was declared to be "cancer free"! We celebrated, had a big party and life was so good. My hair grew in and I actually could get it colored and styled again!

What a thrill that was to be normal again!

I felt good and could do things with my daughter again because I was strong at last. Then, in December of 2013, the unthinkable

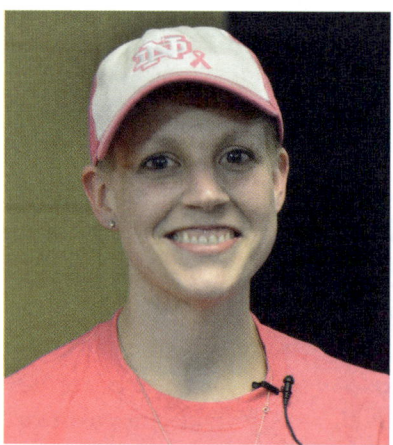
Kendelle Before

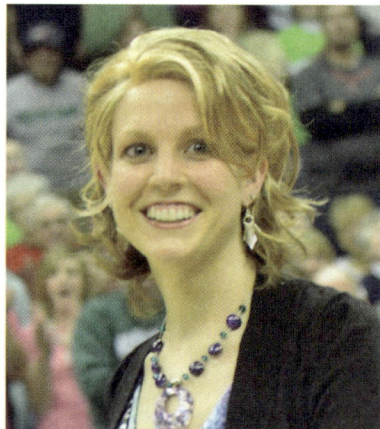
Kendelle After

happened. I found a lump in the area of the first cancer. My oncologist said to check with my plastic surgeon who suggested it could be removed easily and was nothing to worry about. I then visited my regular surgeon who removed the small lump. I waited for the report and once again... "You have cancer" was what I heard.

Now there were more surgeries to get bigger margins! Then it was the treatment plan—what this time? Well, to quote one of my doctors: "We're throwing the kitchen sink at you this time." So I am now doing a different chemotherapy and then radiation, and after that I will have my ovaries removed because my cancer is hormone-driven. I hope that by December 2014, I will once again be "cancer free"!

Despite all of the ugliness of having cancer and all that goes along with it, I have been so fortunate for my family and friends who have been there with me! A very special nurse and friend told me early on that this is just a "blip in time." And she is right. No matter what "blip" happens to me in life, I will meet it head on!

– Kendelle

Tracey's Story
Courage under Fire
(As written by her friend, Julie)

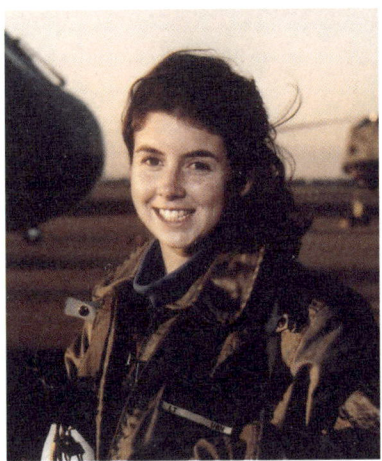

Lt. Tracey Ann Fuchs Yeager
USNA CH-46 Helecopter Pilot,
Norfolk, VA

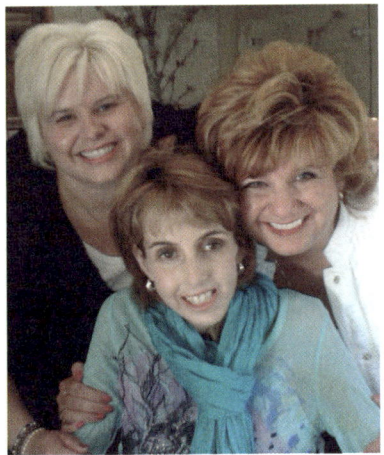

Trisha, Tracey and I
after her makeover

She was my friend, she was vibrant and young. A mother of three beautiful children, a dedicated and loving wife, a woman who had traversed through the mental and physical hardship of graduating from the United States Naval Academy, she flew helicopters, and had served this country. She had conquered more adversities with grace and eloquence than most people I know—and she had stared the cancer devil down five years ago and won. She had been poked, prodded, and surrendered every body part that made her a woman with gratitude—for the promise of life—all the while never wavering in her love of Jesus. She drew strength and composure and optimism from HIM. She held my hand through my own walk with this dreaded disease, and picked me up when I stumbled. So, when I saw her husband, Steve, and dear friend Kevin carrying her down the stairs in a folding canvas chair—the one in which we sat and watched our daughters play soccer, it took my breath away. How could this be? I was suffocating on my own disbelief—My God, I had just seen her three days ago. Now here she was, weak and frail, wincing in pain, and NEVER uttered a complaint. I knew that things were heading toward the path where GOD would be coming to take her home soon. Her body was exhausted, but her spirit was calmly waiting for the Holy Spirit to breathe new life into her—free from cancer. Trying to wrap my head around the whole thing, I secretly wished I had packed a bottle of wine in my bag.

Carried in the chair, too weak to walk, she exhibited the strength and elegance that we all knew her to possess. Carried, yes, but gliding down that red carpet with her head high and taking in the beauty of God's glorious day—as though she were heading down the Royal Red carpet.

Greeted in that Hello Gorgeous! style that comes so naturally to Kim and Trish, we carefully helped her into the mobile DaySpa and settled her in the chair. We laughed because we knew we were going to have some fun. So, with the *Mama Mia* soundtrack booming in the background, the air turned light and exciting, like little girls at their first slumber party. Trac, pronounced Track (as I called her) was up for anything, as usual. She was all about spontaneity and living life, all the while maintaining a humble attitude. She was beautiful inside and out, and today we were going to polish this diamond.

I held her red and swollen legs, where excruciating pain decided to spend the day—legs that had run marathons, had danced with her husband, legs that twirled her children around on the beach, now so painful that they could no longer bear the weight of her 90-pound frame. Trying to find a balance where the pain was tolerable, we traded out ice packs in an attempt to keep the swelling down. She sipped on iced green tea while I resorted to a leftover margarita I scrounged up in her refrigerator. And Trish and Kim worked their magic.

Occasionally I would text Steve that she was fine—but, he was NOT invited to the girlie party—not yet. Patiently he waited in the house. Trish's gentle hands massaged across her forehead, relaxing the pain that she carried in her face and applied a moisture mask. Megan and I gingerly applied lotion and cold packs to her legs, chattering like girls do. Trac joined in, trying not to laugh as the mask tightened on her face. We could see in her breathing when her body hurt, but she pushed through it and laughed with us, reminding us, "It's all good." Her eyes softly closed as she rested. She looked peaceful—finally, a little peace. I discreetly closed the window blinds as I watched car after car pull up for the Reveal. Excitement drowned out the sadness in my heart and the mood turned light.

Softly, Kim matched her skin tone and covered the sores that chemo had decided to leave behind, creating a smooth canvas to skillfully paint a soft palette of makeup. Quiet earth tones began to highlight her bright, sparkly brown eyes. Cancer and its treatment steal the smallest of things one at a time, but we were bringing them back...without cancer's permission.

Highlights were frosted into her hair, as she kept reminding Kim, "Not too much; remember, I like subtle..." and "Nothing too drastic, I want people to recognize me." Trac liked to manage whether she was standing or sitting in a chair. As her hair processed, Trish gently manicured her chemo-damaged nails. I was surprised by the bright red polish she chose. It was bolder than a usual Trac color. I kidded her about the color and she giggled.

Eyes still closed, we could all see that she was getting weary. She was exhausted, and she was in pain. I quietly reached down and pushed Walter—the name she had given the pain pump she had lying on the floor—which was accessed in her port. I never told her, because she would have argued with me that pain meds would weaken her immune system. She was my friend and today was about having fun and being pampered, and the pain medication debate was not up for discussion.

When it came time to rinse the color from her hair, she wrapped her gaunt arms around my neck and I inched her tiny body up from the chair. I remember thinking that I just wanted to take every single moment of being with her into my heart's memory bank. She smelled like lavender, frankincense, and a mixture of essential oils—a smell that I long for on days when the Lord places her on my heart and I see that amazing smile in my mind. She smelled peaceful, as crazy as that sounds. I found a comfort in just being close to her. "Oh, Julie, please go slowly," she murmured, as I lifted and pivoted my feet so she could sit in the chair at the wash basin. I whispered back, "It's okay, I've got you." She had carried me for the last year—keeping my head above water, keeping me focused, keeping me sane in the insanity that cancer brought to my life. It was a gift for me to carry her for a change.

When Kim began to dry her hair, those beautiful golden and auburn highlights that sickness had dulled began to rise like the sun over the autumn-sprinkled lake. She was beautiful. She was radiant. She was ALIVE. When I say "Alive," I mean the Alive that women feel when we slip on a new outfit on our way to a special event. Alive, like when we shut cancer and all of its ugly friends in a closet and slam the door shut—the Alive that comes from our beauty within and explodes on the outside. ALIVE, like when we look in the mirror and there is the reminder of the woman we are on the inside. The Alive seed that Kim and Trish planted, watered, and nurtured all in one short afternoon.

Kim had two outfits that Trac was able to choose from. I helped ease the soft pastel blue and purple chiffon top over her head. The color was perfect! The ocean blue scarf made her beautiful face sparkle with life. Cinching the belt around her tiny waist, we were ready.

I still remember the look on Steve's face as he walked in. I imagined that was the look that he had when he looked down the aisle of the church and saw his beautiful bride waiting to become his wife.

I wondered if this was the look he had when he held each of their children for the first time. Maybe *this* look was that of all of these great moments wrapped in one little package. Or maybe it was the look that he had when he watched her sleep. He saw his beautiful Tracey—the same beautiful Tracey he always saw. Their love filled a room and today it was breaking through the seams of an RV.

Carefully, we carried her to the house where her friends and family had gathered. Like a princess on the top of a cake, Trac sat in the middle of a room where love soared. Trac talked about the day of pampering, saying that it was too much for one girl to take in. Her humility was still at the forefront, as always, as she talked about the wonderful people around her. After about an hour, her friends noticed how very tired she was and they dispersed.

As I placed my lips on her head, I breathed her in; her soft curls tussled in my fingers as I kissed her head and told her that I loved her. I thanked her for the honor of the day, and said that it had been a gift to me to be included. Steve was getting ready to carry her upstairs so she could get some rest.

I called the next day, and he told me that she was so exhausted—but in a good way—that she had been sleeping the whole day. Later that evening, I was typing an article for the local paper about the Hello Gorgeous! girls and their dream to help women feel beautiful in the midst of all of cancer's ugliness. Then, my phone rang.

It was the call that I knew I would get someday, but just didn't think it would be *this* day. God had picked his tired and precious angel from her bed minutes before and carried her home. I called Kim later that night, and we both agreed what an honor and privilege it had been to primp and polish such a beautiful woman to stand face to face with our Lord and Savior, Jesus Himself. It doesn't make it any easier, but somehow it puts a little joy in my heart.

I see her often—in the faces of her children, Samuel, Rachel, and Jack. I see her quirky, crooked smile when I need it the most and I hear her voice always saying "It's all good." Her beauty and elegance is as timeless as the legacy she has left behind. The imprint that Tracey Ann Yeager's short life has left on all of our hearts

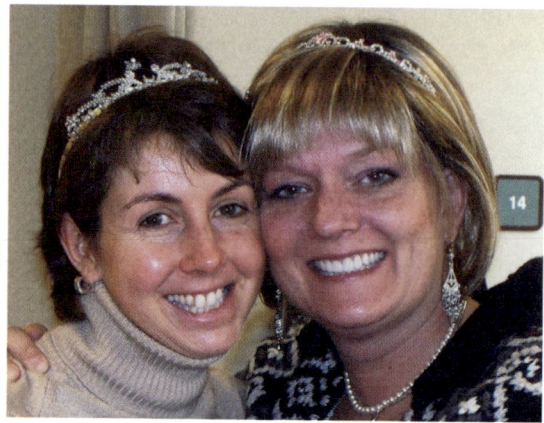

Tracey and Jules

remains constant. Women who have never met her are touched and honored with her award, and it is us and the Hello Gorgeous! Team that will continue to keep her ALIVE—the same Alive I spoke of earlier.

She was my friend, and I will continue to miss her every day.

Lovingly, Jules

Kim Z.
Every Day a Gift

Today, standing on the other side, as an *eleven-year Survivor*, I am grateful for all the *blessings* that have been revealed to me through my cancer journey, which began over eleven years ago in February of 2003, when I discovered a lump in my breast as the result of a breast self-exam.

That same month, on my daughter's fifth birthday, I was diagnosed with Invasive Ductal Carcinoma, HER2+ Breast Cancer. The prognosis was serious. This was an aggressive type of cancer. What happened next can only be described as a tornado ripping through what I used to call my life. My treatment protocol included six months of chemotherapy, surgery, and radiation. The whole process seems so surreal now.

Inspirational Stories < 155

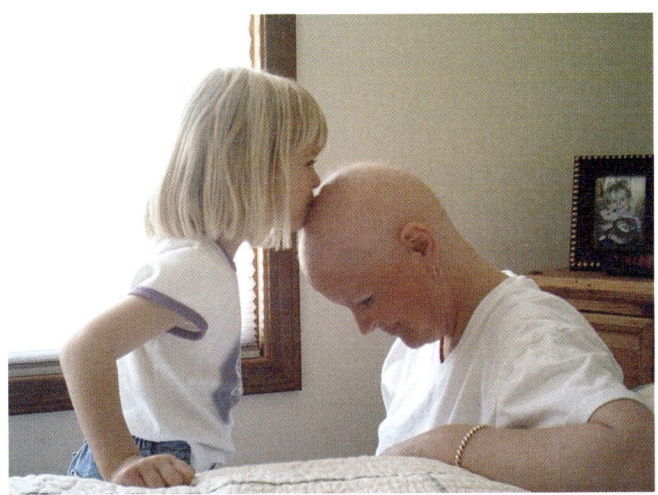

Kim, with her daughter Jordan in 2003

At the same time I was starting my cancer treatment, I was also losing my job of twenty-one years, as the company I had worked for was closing. I lost my hair, my job and my insurance, but *never* my HOPE! My husband Mike—my constant rock—my daughter Jordan (who was only five at the time), and our family and friends were ready to fight! I had too much to live for!

As I was nearing the end of cancer treatment, reality and fear set in. I had cancer! I was not sure what steps to take to move forward with my new life. I really had met only one other young woman when dealing with cancer and pretty much handled the journey myself along with my family. I wish I had known then what I know now. *You do not have to go through this alone!* I am so thankful for my friend who introduced me to a group who was just getting started.

My true healing began when I became involved with the Pink Survivors support group, a group which I now facilitate. These wonderful and inspirational women were facing breast cancer also and had similar issues to those that I was facing as a young woman. The strength that I have gained from my sisters and from our journey together is beyond words. I know they have helped my heart become whole again; and they continue to help me fuel my own personal mission—to help other women get through their cancer journeys.

Today, my life is nothing but a blessing! I am an advocate for others who have to hear the same awful words I did. I have hundreds of Pink friends I call sisters. My career today is: serving the community as a breast-health advocate; helping others find assistance for free mammograms; and, serving as an advocate for those in treatment. I prayed I would see my daughter through grade school. Today she is 16 years old and a sophomore in high school.

My journey has changed me for the better. I try to take the scenic route through life. My heart has opened and allowed me to become an ambassador in the cause, to give back and support those who have to walk the journey that I once did. I am excited to see where my future takes me.

Every day is precious and every breath a gift! – *Kim Z.*

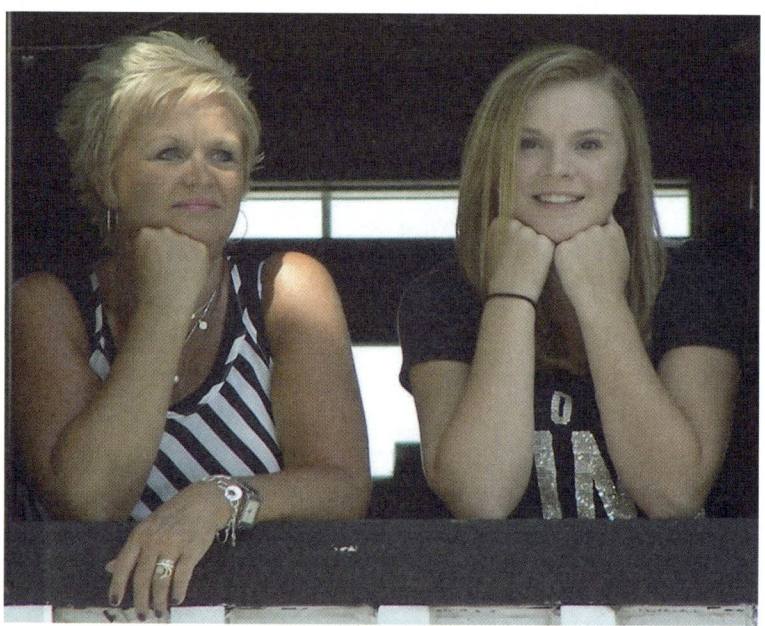

Kim and her daughter Jordan in 2013

Khris and Erin
Hills and Valleys

Life is full of hills, valleys, curves and straightaways. Our family certainly experienced those valleys in 2013, but it was the speckling of hills and sunshine that pulled us through and that I am more excited to share with you now. As I begin, you have to understand that I am really a very private person, so talking about this now feels quite awkward, but we have the hope that our story may in some way help another.

In September of 2012, I underwent a routine mammogram. I don't know about anyone else, but I always have a sense of anxiety going in for the exam, and even more awaiting the results. I was experiencing more anxiety than usual, because my older sister had been diagnosed with breast cancer in 2009, followed by chemotherapy and a mastectomy with reconstruction. My results came back "negative," which was followed by a "whew" moment. "I'm good for another year" (or so I thought). In early December of 2012, I felt a lump in my breast. I not only felt it, but I could see it. I've had calcifications before, but this was different. I tried to convince myself that it was nothing, but knew, in my heart, that this was not going to be good. It was a busy time with work and Holiday planning, but I made an appointment with my gynecologist for December 17th, followed by the mammogram, ultrasound and biopsy on January 2, 2013, with the diagnosis of "Infiltrating poorly differentiated ductal adenocarcinoma"—Triple Negative breast cancer. Not the same as my sister's estrogen-based cancer, but still the dreaded "big C." The journey had begun.

It still amazes me how quickly things happen. I first had to share the news with those close to me. First, a flurry of appointments—the oncologist, an echocardiogram, a PET scan, the surgeon, the genetic counselor, and surgery to have a port put in for the chemotherapy infusions. It quickly became apparent that my life was no longer my own. Cancer was in charge and was dictating my life. Not only was there a medical battle, but now I was going to lose my hair. I was losing the long, thick hair that I had just grown out since my divorce. My "new" image was about to change. Forget the disease that was beginning to spread in my body—I was going to be BALD!

I admire the women who are able to proudly display their bald head with strength and confidence. I know the cancer journey is different for everyone, but this was a tough one for me. Not only did I not want to publicize that I had cancer, but it was an immediate hit to my confidence and vanity. I did not want to be pitied, or for anyone to worry, or for anyone to feel sorry for me. I did not want to be a "victim." In the midst of the medical fog that was occurring, I needed to find a way to maintain "normalcy." I scheduled an appointment for a "wig" consultation—time to prepare for the inevitable.

We continued on the journey. My sister and I sat in the lobby after my appointment with the genetic counselor. I had already strolled through the boutique with the display of wigs, scarves, hats, clothes, creams and other products for persons with cancer. I needed to prepare.

While we sat there I received a phone call that brought me to my knees. A close friend had committed suicide. This was bigger than cancer. She was my friend and I loved her. She had always been a pillar of strength. This could not be happening. The sadness and loss were overwhelming. She had recently emailed me. What had she said in her message? What had I missed? My tears fell and my sister held me.

That evening would be another challenge. I knew that, even with a wig, there would be physical changes that I would not be able to hide. I was hosting the monthly neighborhood Euchre club at my home with many close friends. I would need to tell them. I dreaded sharing my news. I knew that they would all be concerned and want to help, but I didn't want that. I wanted to have this all done and over with. I had already shared the news with my supervisors at work and they extended the news to my coworkers. My request was that the news not be shared with my students and their families. I was already getting more attention than I desired for something that I wanted to go away.

I had the wig consultation and my daughter, Erin, joined in via FaceTime to help me select a wig. In my sister's cancer journey, she had gotten a wig that was even more flattering to her than her natural hair had been and I hoped for the same. That did not occur. I hated them all. I now understood the sadness my sister experienced when she first tried on wigs during her journey. I would look in the mirror and the reflection staring back at me was someone I didn't know. I finally selected a wig that was as close to my own hair as I could find. I walked out with my bag of head covers and hair.

January 18, 2013, was my first chemotherapy appointment. The chemotherapy was going to occur before surgery since it would be a while before the genetic testing results were back that would further direct treatment and surgical options. There would be a total of eight chemotherapy sessions. My sister already knew the routine and the staff. We had bags packed with snacks, books, paperwork and entertainment. I selected a seat near the restroom—a necessity I learned quickly with the infusion of extra fluids and the need to drag an IV pole with me wherever I went. I was given a warm blanket and was set to go. One of the things that I have taken with me from this journey is the strength that I saw in that room. Each person with his/her own story and battle was seated in that room. It certainly didn't feel like a place where someone could feel sorry for oneself. I met so many strong, warm, caring individuals during my journey—including medical staff and other patients—and felt fortunate for that.

I started to lose my hair within a week of the first chemotherapy appointment. I immediately contacted my friend and hairstylist and asked if she would shave my head. She was kind, gracious, and supportive and she agreed. Of course, the hope was that I would be stunning, like Demi Moore in *G.I. Jane*, but that wasn't the case. We cried together as my long hair locks fell to the floor and I again looked at that hated reflection staring back at me in the mirror. I had my wig in tow and I was ready to go. I was having a real issue with my femininity. Little did I know that I would also soon lose my eyelashes, eyebrows and even the hair on my arms. I did not realize how much definition those things add to one's appearance. I was becoming featureless. My arsenal grew to include false eyelashes and an eyebrow pencil. I even ordered a pair of fake eyebrows. They turned out to be big, hairy, scary things. I wasn't looking to be Groucho Marx. I just wanted some definition to my face.

On February 1st we received good news. The BRCA 1 and 2

were negative. I had been so worried that I carried the gene that would impact my entire family for generations to come, but was given some comfort in learning I didn't. I was working, settling into a routine, and things were going fairly smoothly. I was not, however, enjoying trying to get the false eyelashes on each day before work. I would have glue everywhere. I would find my fake lashes coming off during the day like in an old "I Love Lucy" episode, and I could not even figure out where my eyebrows were supposed to go. I was also losing my taste and having digestive issues. Later, I would also experience excessive eye tearing (which really caused a problem with the eyelash application), peeling and swelling of my hands and feet, my fingernails turning dark, and the loss of the majority of my toenails. It would get more and more difficult to maintain that normalcy I so desired.

On February 20th came the next event that would shake our family. Our rescued lab mix, Boomer, had a bump above his eye and was beginning to run into things. He was having difficulty getting in and out of the car and I was becoming weaker from the chemotherapy and had difficulty assisting him. After he had a short hospital stay, we received the devastating news. Boomer had a cancerous brain tumor that was spreading rapidly and had already blinded him. We were going to lose our beloved friend. I brought him home and again had to share our newest tragedy with those who knew him and cared. Marty, a friend and angel, flew in from Alaska to say his good-byes and to support and assist Erin and me with our beloved pet and family member.

In the midst of all of these events, there were also many positive events occurring. There were wedding showers and birthday parties. I was receiving support, encouragement and gifts from coworkers, neighbors, friends and family. There were cards, phone calls, lunch dates and shoulders to lean on. All of these were rays of sunshine that lifted me. I love the human spirit. Life goes on and I was able to celebrate that with others over and over again.

In March came the next tragedy. Believe me, God and I had had a few serious conversations by this point in time, but I always believed and knew He was there with me every step of the way, that there was a plan, and that He would not leave me. My daughter lives a couple hours away and we talk and text often to keep in touch. She had just left a boot camp class and she was sending me pictures of the bruises she had all over her legs and the blood blisters she had in her mouth. She had Googled her symptoms and her research indicated that she should seek immediate medical follow-up. She went to a Med Express clinic and was told that they were going to make an appointment for her to see someone the

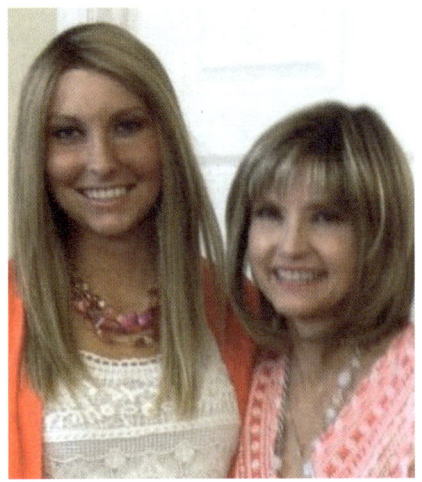

Erin and Khris After

next day. I began researching her symptoms that evening. The next day she called me at work and said that her Dad and I needed to come to the hospital where her appointment was. We were both a couple hours away at the time, but made arrangements to get there as soon as possible. The doctor gave us the shocking news. She was presenting with Acute Promyelocytic Leukemia. The same Leukemia that Chuck Pagano, the Indianapolis Colts' football coach, had battled and won. We were numbed by the news. Was the doctor sure? Couldn't it be some of the less severe diseases that I had read about? What did this mean?

Erin was hospitalized immediately. We would bring the clothes and other things she needed later. Erin doesn't drink or smoke. She works out regularly, played soccer at a Division-I school, and consumes a healthy diet. How could this be happening? They put a treadmill in her room so that she could continue to work out when she felt up to it. She began a treatment of three rounds of intense chemotherapy. She would spend a total of 70 days in the hospital with three bone marrow biopsies, blood transfusions, and a variety of other procedures. We would spend Easter, Mother's Day and Erin's 24th birthday in the hospital. She too would experience the havoc that cancer places on the body. Her head was shaved while in the hospital—more tears and more hugs.

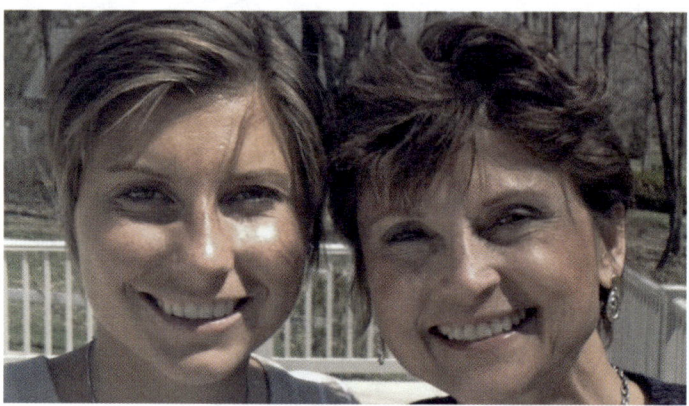

Erin and Khris Now

Though we tried finding a wig, it was too difficult with her in bed most of the time and unable to leave the hospital. She chose to wear scarves and head covers instead. She experienced an acute change in taste, thinning of her lashes and brows, digestive issues and peeling skin. Her body was swollen from the infusions and the steroids. She experienced severe infections, one time ending up in ICU due to an allergic reaction to the preventive antibiotic she had been given. She too had the experience of a strong support system with a stream of gifts, cards, and visitors. Her Dad was there every day for her and made her feel that everything would be okay. He allayed her worries about her job, her bills, her home, the doctors, and what was happening in general. I would stay with her during the weekends that were my off weeks from my own chemotherapy. We would watch TV, talk, paint and otherwise fill the time. Her boyfriend would plan hospital "date nights." Her best friend sent an inspiring, and often humorous, "gift of the day" for a week. She received calls, visits and gifts from family, friends, teammates and her coach. These were the hills among the valleys.

During all that was going on in my life and my daughter's life, my younger sister was trying to plan something special. She had received a flyer on her desk about an organization called "Hello Gorgeous!" and thought it would be perfect for Erin and me. She wanted to plan a special day for us, away from the medical treatments, away from the ugliness of cancer—a day to be pampered, to feel beautiful, and to celebrate a road to recovery. It was to be a surprise. The problem was that we were immersed in treatment and it was difficult to get us both together for a day. Erin eventually had a break in her treatment and wanted to come home for the weekend. My sister called and told us she was going to pick us up on Saturday morning for something and to not ask questions. We both got dressed, and performed our usual fussy new routines with wigs, eyelashes, makeup, etc. She brought us to Sandy's Hair Salon in South Bend, Indiana, where we were greeted with signs, flowers, candy and a team to provide us a day without care. It was amazing. We had facials; challenging manicures and pedicures as we contemplated what to do about my dark fingernails and lack of toenails; put on makeup (gifting the products to us that were used on us that day); and tried on a variety of clothes that had been selected for us from the generosity of the Dress Barn. They sent me off with a new wig, as well, that replaced my own, which had become ratty and worn. After the pampering, the relaxed, beautified and humbled two of us were whisked off to lunch where we were surprised and greeted by friends and family. What a fabulous day!! The day was so very different from those we both had been experiencing for months. We are forever grateful to the Beckers, Hello Gorgeous!, Sandy's Hair Salon, and Dress Barn for being a grand "hill" among our valleys throughout the year.

That wasn't the end of our journey. There were still three surgeries for me, a severe infection from an insect bite near my surgical site, and therapy to improve such things as range of motion. Erin still is required to continue on a regimen of a chemotherapy drug, but we are both now "cancer free." Erin will be attending graduate school in the fall and I will get back to my future plans. We have many new friends from our experiences, lost a few friends along the way, have adopted an even healthier lifestyle, and feel forever blessed by those who touched our lives along the way. Thank you to our family, friends and Hello Gorgeous! We love you all. – *Khris*

Grace
As the Name Implies

(Grace is a very special case. She is the only person in our program to date that has been both a Makeover Specialist and a Gorgeous Woman. As a 20-year stylist, Grace has worked on the business end of the chair and had clients come to her battling cancer and the changes in their appearance. But now, she found herself on the other end of both.)

It all started in June, 2010. My boss came to me at my job doing hair and nails at the JC Penney salon. She asked me if I would be willing to donate my time and give a women going through cancer a manicure. I replied with a willful sure.

"Where are we going to do this?" I asked her. She said a woman came to her named Kim Becker, who does makeovers for women with cancer. Without thinking about it, I asked, "When do we start?" She told me it was an ambush makeover. Penny, my boss, said that it would be in a mobile salon that Kim uses for her makeovers. As it was my turn to perform the manicure, I did the best job I could. It was fun and quite emotional to see the transformation from beginning to end. There were tears of laughter and joy in everyone's eyes.

Now, let's skip forward a couple years. It's January 2012 and there I was, sitting in the doctor's office awaiting the confirmation that I had cancer. We all know how things change after hearing those words. Surgery, recovery, and chemotherapy were the three main stages of my life then. The day arrived when my hair started falling out, and I freaked. Being a hair stylist, it was a little ironic for me to have been giving beauty to others for so many years and not seeing it as clearly then as I do now.

After being cancer free, the family decided to go to Florida for a vacation. My husband told me that we should go to JC Penney's to get clothes for our vacation. As we walked into the door nearest to the salon, I wanted to say "Hi" to my co-workers. There, on the floor, lay a flowing, red carpet. I laughed and I thought, "Who is the red carpet for? What celebrity is here?!" All of a sudden, it got really quiet, and all I heard was "HELLO GORGEOUS!" I turned around to see who was behind me. As it turns out, they were talking to me. Kim and Trisha greeted me with flowers and chocolate, every woman's favorite. I turned to my husband, and said "Oh my god. You knew all along, didn't you?" All I got back from him was an affectionate smile and he told me to have a great time.

My dearest friends gave me my pedicure. My other co-workers fixed my wig. Trisha put on my makeup, and picked out a new outfit. Being treated so well and feeling so Gorgeous! made me feel well again.

As the Gorgeous Ambassador to Hello Gorgeous! for 2012, it has been fun and festive. I am humbled by what Kim, Mike, Trisha, and everyone affiliated with Hello Gorgeous! does for women battling cancer. And it is my great honor to pass this on to the next Gorgeous women. – *Grace*

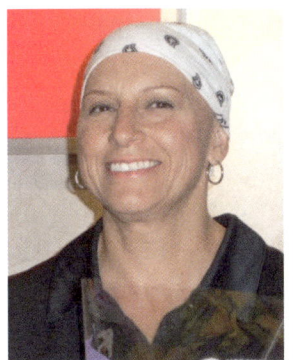
Grace Before

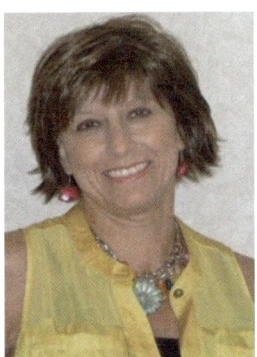
Grace After

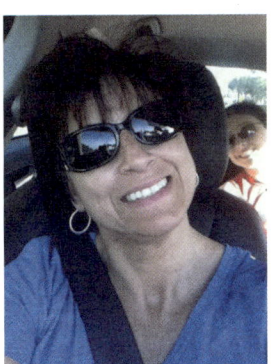
Grace Now

Anne's Story
To Bend, but Not Break

In October of 2011, I had a routine mammogram. A week later I received a letter stating I would need a return visit to check a suspicious area, which came back okay, just fibrous tissue. This had happened twice before but, nevertheless, is nerve-racking, especially recently when a neighbor had gone through a double mastectomy with reconstruction and two co-workers were recently diagnosed. One of my co-workers read a statistic that said three out of ten women that worked together got breast cancer. Hmmm.

In April 2012, I felt an odd-shaped lump in my left breast while taking a shower. Fear, denial, it's just fibrous tissue, maybe a milk duct blockage. A week went by and it started to hurt. Okay, time to see the doctor but should I go to my regular MD or my gynecological nurse practitioner? I opted for my MD who told me he thought it was fibrous, especially since my last mammogram six months ago was okay. I left the office relieved but still had a nagging feeling. Later that week, I went to my gynecologist who also thought it was fibrous. When I came home from that appointment there was a message on my answering machine from my MD telling me that he made an appointment for me to have a follow-up mammogram just to make sure. I debated whether to go or not, but something told me to keep the appointment. On Good Friday, while my family was in church, I was having a mammogram, ultrasound, and needle biopsy—and panic was setting in. How was I going to get through Easter weekend? On Monday I got a call from my MD asking me to come into his office that day. He told me he was very sorry but that it was cancer; Invasive Ductal Carcinoma with several lymph nodes involved. He scheduled me to have a consultation with an oncologist and surgeon later that week at the Elkhart Clinic. He and his staff would pray for me.

I sat in the parking lot and cried, then I called my husband and went back to work. The girls at work would help me, I thought, they would know what to do. We have been through this before in our group. That night telling my son and two daughters was difficult to say the least. After a good cry I asked God to help me get through this and show me the best path to take for His healing, and He did. The rest of the week is a bit of a blur—doctor consultations, blood work, MRI, PET scan. Even though the doctors at the Elkhart Clinic gave me a good prognosis, I got a second opinion at Goshen Cancer Center.

I immediately felt a calm there when I walked through the doors. My husband and I spent the day meeting my oncologist, surgeon, nutritionist and psychologist. It was to be 20 weeks of chemo, surgery, and then 36 days of radiation, followed by reconstruction. It was a lot to take in for one day. Goshen had the same prognosis as the Elkhart Clinic; however, I felt a peace here. During Mass one Sunday, as I asked God if Goshen was the right decision, the surgeon I had consulted with in Goshen came walking down the church aisle. I never even knew he was a member of our church! God was telling me—this is where you need to be.

My neighbor brought me books to read when my mind raced with anxiety like hers did. She also told me many hints to use to get through chemo, like: eating with plastic silverware because everything will taste like metal, and using a numbing cream on my port site before the infusion so the needle stick isn't so bad. My co-workers also gave me such great tips, such as a rinse to use a few days prior to treatment to help with mouth sores. They brought my family meals on the day of my chemo. I will be forever grateful for all their support.

Then I called Kim. I have known Kim since she was four years old and she has been cutting my hair for close to 25 years. In 2005, she told me of a "vision" she had of helping women going through cancer treatment; giving them makeovers and traveling all over the country doing this. At the time I thought she had LOST HER MIND! Now here I was, needing her skilled care. How ironic. Losing my hair did not worry me because I knew Kim would take care of me. By the grace of God, Hello Gorgeous! had become such an amazing support system for women.

On April 27, 2012, I began my first chemo treatment. As I sat in the infusion room, I remembered a conversation Kim and I had when she first began her journey with Hello Gorgeous! She would tell me about the women she had met during her first makeovers and how much inspiration and conviction she received. She also found that women deal with their diagnosis in very different ways; some became PINK warriors, while others went through the treatment and went on with their lives as if it never happened. My oncologist told me, "Don't let cancer define who you are." I wondered what kind of survivor I would be, and I *WAS GOING TO SURVIVE!!*

Chemo was not fun, but there were folks I met during treatment that blessed me in so many ways. They gave me hope, love, and encouragement. I met a woman who was going through treatment for the third time. We would sit next to each other every week and share symptoms, home remedies to feel better, and many laughs. We lifted each other up and encouraged others to keep their spirits up as well. I will forever keep them in my prayers.

After the third infusion, my hair started to fall out. I could run my hand through my hair and handfuls would come out. It kind of fascinated me. A few weeks earlier Kim had cut my natural hair to match the style of wig she found for me, so that the transition would be smooth. And it was. Not even my husband noticed that anything was different.

May 19, 2012, was the day of Penn High School's prom. I was sitting watching from a chair as Kim and her sister, Trisha, did both of my daughters' hair in updos. Kim looked over and smiled.

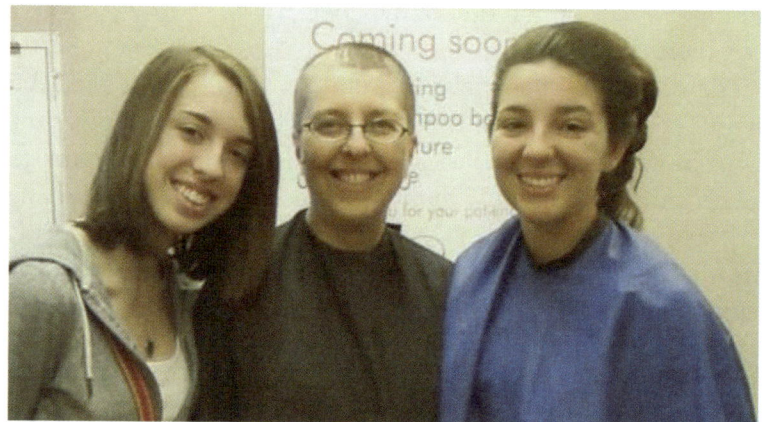

Anne and Daughters on Prom Day

"How's your hair doing?" I whipped off my wig and we both smiled at each other and said, "It's time." I sat in Kim's chair as she shaved my head, CRYING FOR ME, and I comforted her.

"It's only hair, it will grow back." God love Kim. As my daughters watched, Kim shaved my head. I made up my mind that I was going to show my daughters that cancer was a journey that had some unpleasant aspects, but with God's help, "We might bend, but we won't break."

In September 2012, my left breast and 36 lymph nodes were removed. I decided NOT to have both breasts removed and no reconstruction. The surgery went smoothly and I actually came home that same day. I felt good. It was weird but, as far as I was concerned, the cancer was out of my body. I would go shopping, looking at ruffled shirts, thinking that no one would notice I was lopsided. And even if they did, who cares? It was more important for me to show my daughters that women are more than boobs. For quite a while, I did not use a prosthetic breast (or chicken cutlet as we like to call it). One day a patient in the dental office I worked at encouraged me to take off my wig and "Let it go!!" My hair was peach fuzz and a little curly, but I was okay with myself. I will not let my breasts or lack of hair define who I am.

On October 17, 2012, I was surprised with a HELLO GORGEOUS! Makeover. My co-workers and family had kept this secret for almost a month. The front door at my office opened with Kim shouting, "HELLO GORGEOUS!" I did not feel worthy of such a fabulous day. I had seen so many other women during my treatment who were so much more deserving than myself. But here I was, being whisked away in a limo with a red carpet, champagne, flowers and chocolate. A few minutes later, I was at FIX Salon/Spa getting pampered. I had my first facial, which was divine, and a manicure and pedicure. The Makeover Specialists brought out several outfit options, one with a pair of RED pants. Normally I'm pretty boring with my clothes, so I decided to be sassy and chose the red pant outfit. They did my makeup, washed and styled my wig, and Kim did the finishing touches. I felt GORGEOUS! Then, back in the limo and off to lunch, where my family and friends were waiting at my surprise Reveal. I cried. I still do when I look at the pictures. Words cannot express how wonderful that day was for me. Kim has made me eat my words about her "crazy idea" from so many years ago.

Soon after my makeover, I began 36 days of radiation, and continued Herceptin infusions for a year. The radiation was a bit daunting, with that huge machine hanging over you. My son and I are Star Wars fans, so I would envision Jesus with a light saber zapping the remaining cancer cells away. It was during one of my treatments that I truly felt His hand on my left side healing me. "The hurt and the Healer collide."

Thanks also to all the "helpful hints" I received from Kim and

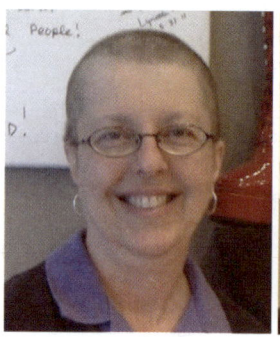 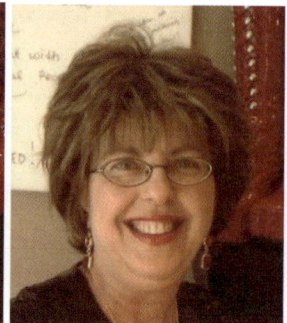 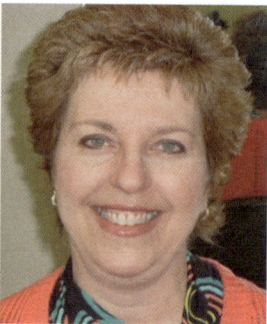

Anne Before   Anne After   Anne Now

friends who had gone through the same treatments. I started to burn only about a week before my last radiation. I had my last cancer treatment on my daughter's birthday. I do not take any medication and when I asked my oncologist what the next step in my treatment was, he told me "to live a long and happy life." That's what I intend to do, PRAISE GOD!!!

It has been two years. What kind of survivor am I? Still working on that one. I would love to put a book together for folks going through chemo and radiation—the side effects and helpful hints you learn from others who have already been there and done that! I have also been honored to help Kim with a HELLO GORGEOUS instructional video on "My hair's growing back. How do I style it?" God has blessed me with family and friends who have supported me. He has blessed me with healing and He has blessed Kim and Mike as well. It is truly their calling. We are all beautiful, we are HELLO GORGEOUS! – Anne

Tina's Story
A Sister's Story

I had just turned 40 and had been having female problems for a while, but I hadn't contacted my doctor yet. I told my sister Amy about the problems I had been having and she started calling me *every day* to see if I had made a doctor's appointment yet. I finally made an appointment, but it seemed like every time the new date came up I would be bleeding. I began spotting the morning of my next appointment but decided to keep it. The doctor was glad I had come in.

It had been a long time since my last pap test and he said I would get the results by mail in about a week if everything was all right. The next Friday I missed a call from his office and, when I returned the call, I found out that the doctor had called me himself. I knew I was in trouble at that point. He told me that I had abnormal cells show up and we had to do some biopsies. I started to cry and he said that it was probably nothing.

The following week my husband and I went to his office for the tests. I was bleeding too much, so I needed to have a DNC. That next Friday we went in for the DNC and, after it was over, the doctor had already told my husband that, at the very least, I would have to have a full hysterectomy. But it looked to be a benign tumor.

On June 22, 2012, I got the call that no one ever wants to get. I answered the call at work and the doctor said that he hated giving this kind of news over the phone, but I said that I just wanted to know. He said, "You have cancer," and that he had to refer me to a specialist.

I don't remember anything after the words, "You have cancer."

I got off the phone and told my boss, "I have cancer," and that I needed to leave to tell my husband. I called my sister Amy and told her that I had cancer and that I had to see a different doctor. I called my sister Kim crying and told her I have cancer. I had to get home and tell Sean.

When I got home, Sean came running up to tell me that everything was going to be all right. I told him, "This is your out. I can't give you the children that you want but someone else can." He said he wasn't going anywhere and that we would get through this together. It was shut-down time at the company I worked for, so Sean and I were scheduled to leave town for just over a week. I got ahold of the oncologist's office, not knowing what to do, but they said to go out of town and they would see me when we got back.

It was a restless vacation. My Aunt Sue had been sick and had just come home from the hospital the week before. As we headed back to Indiana, I wanted to hurry to her. It was then, while we were still on the road, that Sean received a call telling us that my favorite aunt had died. They had found her that morning in bed. I was so upset! I found myself so mad at her for leaving me!

So that next week was my first visit with my cancer doctor…and my Aunt's funeral services. It was all happening too fast. We found out that all three biopsies came back positive, that I needed a radical hysterectomy, that he might be able to get all the cancer that way, and that it needed to be done soon.

On August 6, 2012, I went into the hospital for surgery. Afterwards, the doctor came in to let us know that he got it all. When we went to my follow-up appointment, we found out that I had a very rare and aggressive cancer called Neuroendocrine Carcinoma of the cervix. I would have to go through four rounds of chemo and that they would have to hit me as hard as was medically allowed. The first thing I asked was if I was going to lose my hair. He said maybe. I started to cry.

I started chemo in October. The regimen was to be three days on chemotherapy, then 18 days off. That was one round. We had a plan in place if my hair started to fall out and, two weeks after my first chemo treatment, I got in the shower and started to wash my hair. The next thing I knew, I had two hands full of hair. I called Kim and said that tonight was the night. I told Sean that I was having my head shaved that night. He plays poker on Wednesdays and I told him to go and I would be fine. I didn't realize that it was going to hurt so bad when it started falling out. It feels like thousands of needles in your head.

We had a little party there—my Mom, my sisters, two friends and me. Amy was going to get her head shaved too, but I asked her not to. Why should she look sick? So she got her hair cut very short. I cried when we started buzzing my head. I couldn't look in the mirror. Kim had three wigs for me that we cut and styled.

I had a couple cute knit hats that Kim had given me. I decided to wear one to the store to get a script filled and do some shopping. I have never had so many people stare at me and make me feel so bad. I sat in my car and texted my sisters crying, "Why are people so mean? They stare at sick people and make them feel worse than they already do."

My nephew Joe had some teeth pulled that day so I went to sit with him until Amy got home. I didn't want to sit around alone and feel sorry for myself. All of a sudden Amy was home, my mom was at the door, and Kim and Trish weren't far behind. They decided to surprise me with a new look—big, fun earrings, new makeup, and a "Live Strong" hat. I found the wigs to be hot and itchy and preferred a bandana or a hat. After that great experience, I decided to have the new attitude of, "Shame on you for staring at me!" and to hold my head up high!!! The next day when leaving chemo, my mom and I went into the boutique at the treatment center and found a teal hat that said: "Fight Like a Girl!" So that is what I did.

We were planning a trip to Las Vegas in April of 2013 with Sean's family and I found out that there was a conference called "Stupid Cancer" there at the same time. So I signed up to attend it and the classes it offered.

The weekend before we left for Vegas, we were supposed to open our trailer for the season. I told Sean I didn't want to go until after Vegas, but he said there was a new golf cart he wanted to look at and go to dinner at Joe's Crab Shack in Fort Wayne. So we went down and spent the night Saturday and he said he wanted to attend the lot owners meeting, which we never do, so we went. As the meeting started and the door opened, in came my whole family with the Hello Gorgeous! banner and my surprise visit! It was a wonderful day of pampering and love, all for me. I cried and could not believe they had got me! And the new outfit was perfect for my Las Vegas trip.

So we were at dinner our first night in Las Vegas with all these women from across the United States with my same cancer and one of my cancer sisters asked if I knew this person who had approached our table. When I turned around, there stood Kim. I started to cry and asked what she was doing there. She said she was there to take classes with me. The next thing I knew, in comes my mother and my other sisters carrying a "love and support" banner for me that they had all signed. I couldn't believe they were all there. My three sisters and I were going to classes together.

Amy had done some research and found a Facebook page entirely of women that had my same kind of cancer. I could go to this page and ask any questions that I wanted and nobody looked at you funny. Everyone there had been through it, or were still going through it. These are my sisters from another mother, I thought. I learned to love these women and cannot thank them enough!!! We Are Rare but There.

I made it through the rest of chemo well. The last round was the worst. I have to thank my husband Sean, his family and my family, for making sure that I was never alone for anything through all of this. I am now one and a half years cancer free—and plan to stay that way! – *Tina*

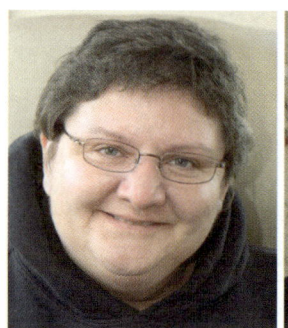
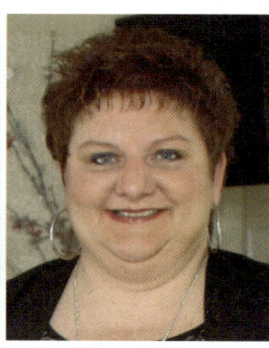
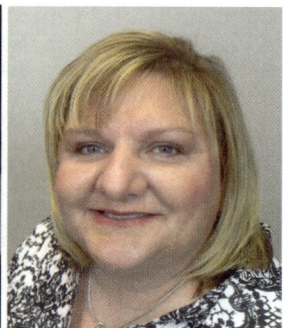

Tina Before   Tina After   Tina Now

Deb
Four Years and Counting

About four years ago, I was feeling great. I was working for Weight Watchers, trying to be as healthy as I could. It came time for my mammogram and I thought to myself that I probably will not go and have it done because I felt wonderful. But my husband said to just go and have it done because all the other mammograms were okay. Just get it done.

I made my appointment and got the test done. I remember like it was yesterday when they came back to me and told me that they thought they saw something. They wanted to do another test. I thought maybe they just wanted to use up my insurance. I agreed and this time things were a bit more serious. They had definitely found something and I would need a biopsy. During the biopsy, I could feel through the people around me that it was not good, but no one said a word.

It seemed like a long time before I found out from my doctor that it was true. I really did have breast cancer. I couldn't believe that it was me! I think I went into a different place in my head. My doctor put me on stronger antidepressants and we headed to the cancer center. That was the day that we found out what I was going to have to do to get well.

They gave us this bag with all kinds of goodies and told us about the chemo treatments, and after that would come the radiation. But first, I had to have surgery to remove the cancer. After surgery, the chemo began. Every three weeks! My doctor informed me that I would lose my hair the first month of chemo, but I thought I would be different.

By the end of the first month, my hair was coming out in clumps. So my husband and I decided to go ahead and shave it off. My husband was ahead of me in this game—he had ordered a wig that pretty much matched my hair. So, for a while, everyone thought it was my own hair. After six months of chemo, I was informed I would have 33 radiation treatments. I wasn't going to do it, because I thought the chemo should have been good enough. But the doctor told me that the kind of cancer I had was very aggressive and I should do it all, just to make sure it was gone. At least I hoped so.

After my last treatment I received a wonderful treat. My good friend and office manager had secretly nominated me for a Hello Gorgeous! visit at FIX Salon/Spa in Elkhart. That day was so amazing! I got the royal treatment—I had my hair cut and colored (what little I had!), a facial, a manicure and my toes done. I got new clothes, flowers and candy, plus a dinner afterwards with all my friends and family.

I loved everything about this day, but I couldn't help but feel guilty about getting all that pampering, because I knew there were a lot of other women who were a lot sicker than I was. I would not have had this wonderful day were it not for the wonderful people of Hello Gorgeous! Those people donate their time and money to make our day absolutely perfect.

I want to add that my life has been changed—my outlook and my faith. God has been very good to me and I know He gave me this time to be there for others. And if my story helps even a little, then I have done something to give back. I am now four years…and counting! – *Deb*

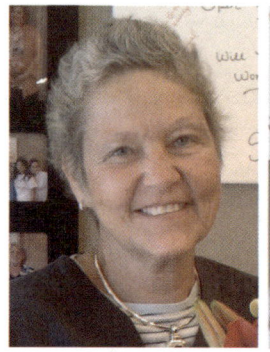 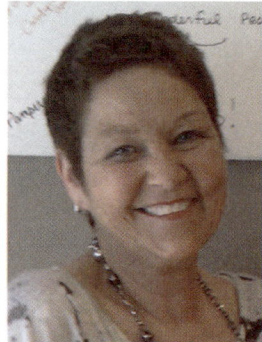 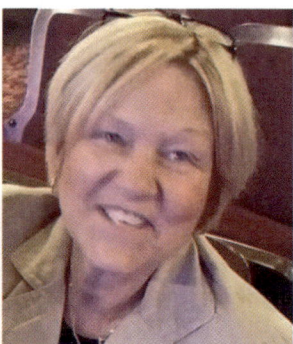

Deb Before   Deb After   Deb Now

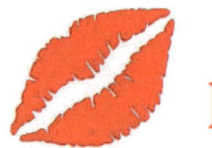 ## K.I.S.S. Tip

Test new products on the inside of your wrist 24 hours before using it on your whole body. Choose mild products specifically formulated for sensitive skin.

*"Life isn't about finding yourself.
It's about creating yourself."*
– George Bernard Shaw

Chapter 15

Stories from the Affiliates

Our Salon Affiliates are selfless salon owners and stylist teams that use their stellar talents to perform the Hello Gorgeous! Experience on women battling cancer in their communities across the United States. They are certified by Hello Gorgeous! of HOPE and perform these ambush makeovers on members of their own communities each month. And they will tell you, as Mike and I will, that what they receive from working with these amazing, Gorgeous Women, is more than they could ever give to them.

These are a few of the stories from our Affiliate Salons about the women they serve who have changed their lives forever.

> "Never believe that a few caring people can't change the world.
> For, indeed, that's all who ever have."
> – Margaret Mead

Julene
FIX Salon/Spa

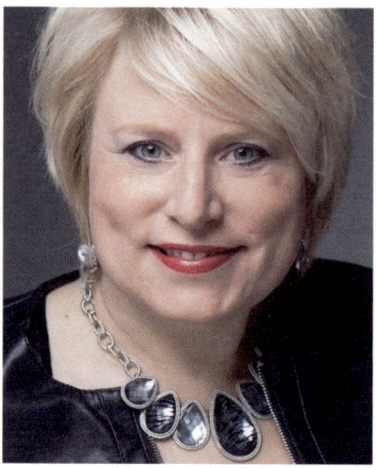

In thinking back over the many makeovers at my salon, in regards to the clothing, something that has stood out for me is that many women are feeling so empowered on that day of their makeover because they are so excited to try on new styles of clothes that they would never have picked out for themselves. One of my Gorgeous Women even tried on a pair of red pants! She said, "I would NEVER buy myself a red pair of pants." Well, guess what?! Those were the ones that she chose! She said that she had never felt so sassy and gorgeous before! So, just because a woman, walking the journey of cancer, "always" wears sweat pants and a t-shirt does not mean that she "loves" wearing sweatpants and a t-shirt. When you give a red-carpet makeover experience, these women want to look like they belong there.

When first becoming a Hello Gorgeous! Salon Affiliate, I received a call from the nominator of the Gorgeous Woman that we were surprising that day. They were on their way to the salon, but she wanted to give me a "heads up"—the nominee was on morphine and in a lot of pain. I felt a bit panicked, hearing that news, so I called Kim Becker immediately, asking what to do. Kim's advice was perfect. She told me to go ahead with the makeover but to let our woman know that at any time during the services, if she felt uncomfortable or needed to stop, to just say so. Kim also reminded me that, many times, these women start feeling better as they experience such a great day focused on them. And Kim was absolutely right! This woman relaxed fully about halfway through her facial, somehow finding a renewed level of energy, and felt much better. It was a BIG "aha" moment for me to see that kind of positive impact firsthand—going from a woman who, in the beginning, could barely make it through our front door, to one who was looking gorgeous and striking a pose three hours later!

The ongoing effects of the Hello Gorgeous! Experience has been HUGE for me. I cannot tell you how many family members, months later, have told me (tearfully) what that day meant for their loved one and for them. One of our salon guests, who was also one of our Hello Gorgeous! Makeover recipients, still talks about that day to me when she comes in for her regular salon appointments—two years later! She continually says to me, "You just DO NOT know the impact of that day for me."

Of course, some of these dear women lose their battle and I attend their funeral. It has been another reminder of the effects of the Hello Gorgeous! Experience, when I find her laid to rest in the outfit she received the day of her makeover. It touches me deeply to see her wearing the outfit that she felt so Gorgeous in and that her family chose for her final outfit.

This experience is so much more than one day in a woman's life. It affects more than just the woman herself. Many times it is the "bright spot" in their journey...and the light that shines bright enough for them to walk forward. And when they look back over their journey, they see that light—a reminder—that it was not ALL dark for them during that time. It fills my heart to the brim.

> Julene Melendez
> Owner, FIX Salon/Spa
> Elkhart, Indiana

Sandy
Sandy's Hair Design

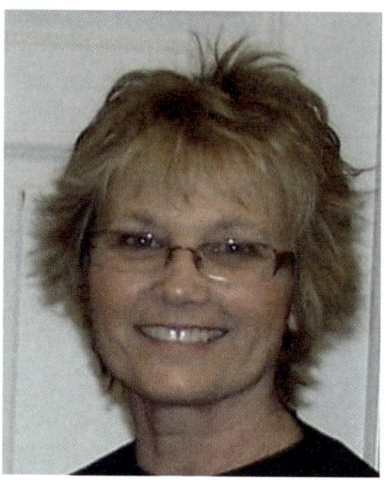

(Sandy's Hair Design was our first Affiliate Salon. We refer to Sandy's as our "First Born." It was very much because of meeting Sandy Zanka, and experiencing her overwhelming passion and drive to help these women battling cancer, that Mike and I have worked so hard to build this program. To this date, Sandy and her crew have done over 50 makeovers on women in her community. She holds a fashion show and luncheon fundraiser each year for her Affiliate, where she brings back all of her Gorgeous Women as her models for the show. She does not realize how much this program owes her and her efforts, and we just wanted to thank her and her girls for their selfless work. God Bless, Sandy!)

Being a Hello Gorgeous! Affiliate Salon, I am often asked which Hello Gorgeous! visit has impacted us the most. Each visit and each woman is unique in their own way. With some, you are amazed by their faith, some with their courage, and some with their humor. And also, in some circumstances, you are taken aback by their loss. I truly feel that I would somehow minimize the other ladies we have served if I said that there was one that stood out above the others. Each and every story touches you in so many dimensions. So I guess my answer would be my very first visit.

Her name was Diane and she was the beginning for us. She

opened the door to my salon and gave my staff and me this fabulous gift that has kept on giving. Since Diane's visit, we have done over 50 visits in our salon. And starting in October of 2010, we have been fortunate enough to be in this program for three and a half years.

To see them walk into my salon, help to breathe life back into them, and then to see them dance out, it makes me realize that what we do is truly a gift from God.

> Sandy Zanka
> and Staff at Sandy's Hair Design
> South Bend, Indiana

Dana
Creative Edge Hair Studio

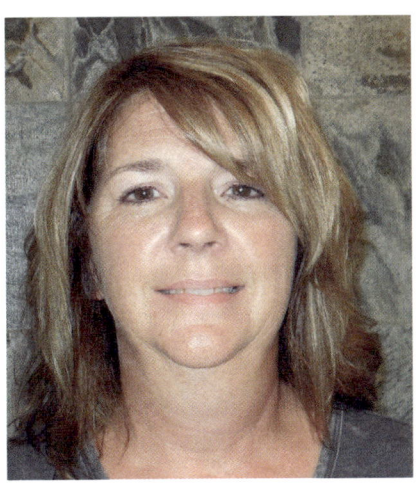

My story is about my own Aunt Susie. She has been battling pancreatic cancer for about a year now. Once she was nominated by Hello Gorgeous! and her nomination came to us, we surprised her at her home with a limo. She was reluctant to go, saying she didn't need this special treatment and to save it for someone else. But we would not take no for an answer!

She told us that she had the best day ever! She was so glad she had come. But the impact on me was profound. We have been with Hello Gorgeous! as an Affiliate Salon for three years and every experience has been amazing. But when it is a personal relationship, it really hits home. To see my Aunt go from simply defeated to "I want to conquer the world" was such a blessing! I can still see the smile on her face through the whole experience. Just putting on makeup again after everything she has been through made her feel beautiful!

She fought us on taking the new outfit, saying that she didn't deserve it or need the clothes, but she truly did, not having bought a thing after losing so much weight. I was extremely touched! She then got the biggest surprise of all when her whole family was waiting at our local Logan's Roadhouse for dinner. I feel so incredibly blessed to be a small part of Hello Gorgeous! of HOPE because that's what it does—it brings Hope to these special, deserving women!

I was so overwhelmed driving home that evening after her makeover that I cried the whole way home, for many reasons—for my Aunt and what she has been through; for being able to share it with my other aunts, uncles, and cousins; and I especially felt blessed to be a part of this organization.

Thank You! Thank You! Kim and Mike for letting me and my girls be a small part of your journey. What a gift you are! :)

> Love,
> Dana
> Creative Edge Hair Studio
> Mishawaka, Indiana

Leeca

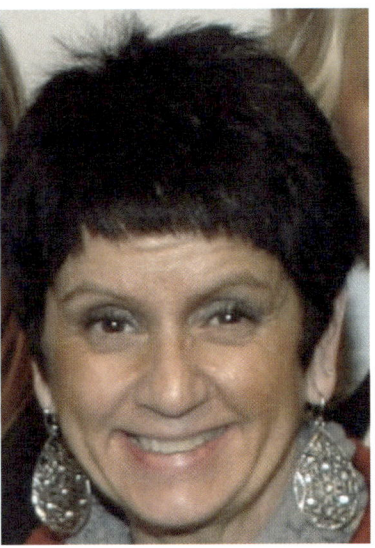

A Profound Effect

(Leeca is the manager of a Maurice's store in the Indianapolis area who has the ultimate passion for Hello Gorgeous! and our women. Her efforts have led to a relationship between us and Maurice's locations in cities across the United States. Leeca is one in a million!)

I would like to share with you something that happened to me over the weekend. It has made me realize how lucky I am to work for a company that encourages us to help our fellow man. I feel very fortunate being associated with Hello Gorgeous! and I feel there is so much we do with this organization that impacts so many women as well as the lives of many who are associated with them. I would like to let you know what our contributions bring to the women who have been a part of a Hello Gorgeous! event.

Back in February, we did a Hello Gorgeous! makeover for Linda. Linda was a customer in my store. She had been coming into the store regularly, buying some things, but mostly coming in for the socializing that we naturally do with our customers. Linda had cancer and would share with us her worsening condition and some of the hardships she was having. It dawned on me that I should nominate her for a makeover. So it took some doing, but we were able to contact her sister Pam to help us surprise Linda. We partnered with Chateau Bijou and provided a lovely afternoon of pampering and fellowship for Linda. Her two sisters, Pam and Cassie, were with her all the way and I was lucky to be able to stay with them as well because I had the day off. I got to know these women and I felt like I was part of their family. Linda got her makeover and she looked so beautiful with her makeup done, wearing her new wig and her brand new outfit.

As the months progressed, Linda's condition worsened—although she actually lived long past the time her doctors had given her. Linda passed away last Wednesday, which was a blessing because of the great pain and suffering she had been enduring. Her sister Cassie had let me know. I decided that I should go pay my respects to Linda and her family. Pam and Cassie were very glad I showed up and they introduced me to Linda's immediate family.

The purpose of this story is to let you know how the things we do in our stores have an effect on our customers and ourselves. I was very moved to find out that pictures of the makeover day were in Linda's memory book and that a picture of me giving Linda flowers was on a monitor displaying pictures of Linda's life. It was very moving and I cherish the fact that I was able to provide that memory for Linda and her sisters and it obviously meant something to them as well. We always hear from customers the effect we have on them, but I just wanted to let you know that it has had a profound effect on me and my team also, that we were able to do this for Linda. And it's because Maurices allowed us to do it.

Leeca,
manager
Maurices

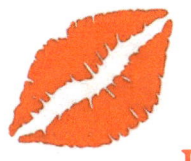

K.I.S.S. Tip

Apply your foundation—liquid, cream, or powder—and then gently push the product into your skin with small circular motions with your tool of choice. It should look and feel as if it's melted in, instead of just spread on top.

> *"Don't judge each day by the harvest you reap, but rather by the seeds you plant."*
>
> – Robert Louis Stevenson

The Journey Continues

So that's it. Mike and I did not want to make this a complicated, thousand-page manual that would intimidate you from the start. We kept it small, friendly, and easy to use.

We have tried to give you enough information in each area to allow you to look your best in the worst situation. We have included videos for the complicated areas, and have given you amazing, inspirational stories of women just like yourself—women living their lives in the face of this danger with strength and will and grace and fear, but with the resolve to face the fear. And we have told you about the noble and talented people of the Affiliate Program who help our women battling cancer to pick themselves up and always remember that there are people in the world who still care for others. But there is one more thing.

In our first book, *Hello Gorgeous! A Journey of Faith, Love and Hope*, I introduced my sisters to you. They are all very important to me. And so when I began this Calling, my Hope was that I would never have to use this knowledge and these services for

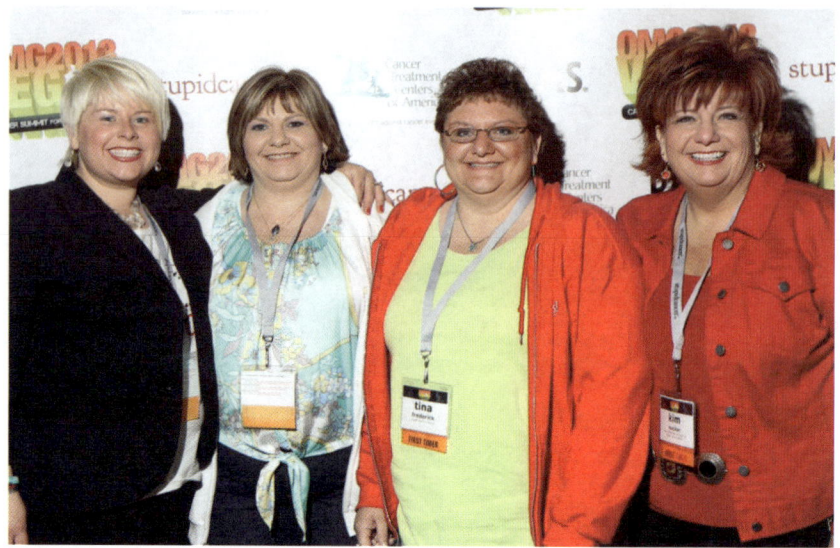

The Sisters: Trisha, Amy, Tina and Kim

any of them. Well, God had other plans. But I am so very grateful that I have the knowledge that helped my sister Tina through her cancer journey, and that now I can help every woman who has been diagnosed with cancer and who needs this information to stay Red-Carpet Gorgeous!

So, I hope you reach your "there." And I hope you put your lipstick on when you get there.

God Bless!

"Our deepest fear is not that we are inadequate. Our deepest fear is that we are powerful beyond measure. It is our light, not our darkness that most frightens us. We ask ourselves, Who am I to be brilliant, gorgeous, talented, fabulous? Actually, who are you not to be? You are a child of God. Your playing small does not serve the world. There is nothing enlightened about shrinking so that other people won't feel insecure around you. ... We were born to make manifest the glory of God that is within us. It's not just in some of us; it's in everyone. And as we let our own light shine, we unconsciously give other people permission to do the same. As we are liberated from our own fear, our presence automatically liberates others."

– Marianne Williamson

Material Lists

Finger Nails
Cotton balls
Hand lotion
Cuticle oil
Fingernail polish remover
Orangewood stick
Fingernail file
Base coat
Top coat
Nail color

Toes
Cotton balls
Foot lotion
Fingernail polish remover
Orangewood stick
Pumice stone
Fingernail file
Base coat
Top coat
Nail color

Human-Hair Wig Care

Wig shampoo or professional salon shampoo
Wig conditioner or professional salon conditioner
Bath towel
2-liter pop bottle
Wig stand or Styrofoam head

As needed to style your Human-Hair wig the way you like

Brush
Blow dryer
Curling iron
Flat iron
Hot rollers

Synthetic-Hair Wig Care

Wig shampoo
Bath towel
2-liter pop bottle
Wig stand or Styrofoam head
Brush
Wig hairspray, if needed

Makeup

Cotton balls
Cotton swabs
Makeup sponge

Skin Care

Disposable washcloth
Cotton balls
Disposable makeup spatulas

Glossary of Terms

Acetone Polish Remover – a type of polish remover that contains acetone, a solvent used as an ingredient in some paint thinners and cleaning supplies. This type of nail polish remover usually takes off nail polish easier than one that does not contain this ingredient. It is also useful for taking off false nails and removing strong glue from fingers.
Acrylic Nails – false nails that are fastened to your natural nails to give them a longer look. This is not a process we recommend for a woman going through cancer.
Base Coat – a clear coat that acts as a primer in nail painting. In most cases, it is a basic clear nail polish, though some brands offer base coats with protein, aloe vera, vitamin E, and the like. These featured ingredients add strength and resiliency to the nail.
Blush – red or pink makeup in powder or cream form used to add color to the cheeks or to accentuate the shape of the cheekbones.
Certified Makeover Specialist – a licensed cosmetologist who has been certified in the Hello Gorgeous! Experience, and understands the cosmetic service precautions that should be taken with a woman battling cancer.
Chemotherapy – the use of chemical agents or drugs to treat diseases, infections, or other disorders, but to most people chemotherapy refers to drugs used for cancer treatment. These drugs can change your physiology and severely lower your immune system, which is why we suggest simple precautions when receiving cosmetic services during your treatment.
Cleanser – a facial cleanser that, in the broadest application, is a cleaning agent used to remove a buildup of dirt, grime, or oil from your face. These products are used to remove makeup from the skin, allowing the pores to breathe and complete cleansing of the face to occur.
Concealer – makeup for hiding blemishes; flesh-colored makeup that can be applied to the skin to hide blemishes.
Conditioner – a hair care product that is applied after shampooing in order to condition the hair. It is most useful for people with dry or damaged hair to restore moisture and to smooth the cuticles of the hair follicles. Again, professional products found at prominent hair salons are always recommended over less expensive retail store brands for the integrity of your hair.
Cotton Ball – A cotton ball is made from natural cotton fibers, which are processed and shaped into round balls that are typically white in color. Be-

cause of its shape, appearance, and ability to absorb liquids, cotton balls have a variety of uses for manicures, pedicures, makeup and skincare.

Cotton Swab – found at any drug, grocery or discount store, cotton swabs are plastic or paper sticks with small cotton-wrapped ends usually reserved for cleaning your ears. These make wonderful makeup tools and allow you to dispense product from a container, in a sanitary way, without using your finger and risking contamination.

Curling Iron – a heated rod for curling hair; a device consisting of a heated rod around which the hair is twisted to form a curl.

Cuticle Oil – a moisturizing product used in nail care. Made from various types of oils, it is designed to be applied with a brush, cotton ball, or pen on the cuticles—the small, slightly hardened strip of skin at the base of the fingernails and toenails.

Dry Shampoo – a popular alternative to regular shampoo in recent years. It absorbs the oil that makes your hair look greasy without drying your scalp out, like washing your hair with water every day can do.

Emery Board – pieces of cardboard, which have emery or emery paper glued to them, making them both abrasive and flexible, that are used for fingernail and toenail care.

Eye Liner – a cosmetic for the eyelids, usually applied in a thin line close to the lashes to accentuate the eyes.

Eye Shadow – a colored cosmetic for the area around the eyes, especially the eyelids.

Eyebrow Pencil – a soft cosmetic pencil used to darken the eyebrows.

Facial – a beauty treatment for the face and a very general term for a variety of skin treatments which can include: steam, exfoliation, extraction, creams, lotions, facial masks, and massage, usually performed by a licensed aesthetician.

False Eyelashes – synthetic eyelashes that are worn on top of a person's regular eyelashes to make them look longer and fuller. This is not a process we recommend for a woman going through cancer.

Flat Iron – a hair care product that is used to straighten hair. The iron is heated, usually through a cord that is plugged into the wall, creating a heated surface that, when run over hair strands, heats up the hair follicles and molds them to the desired position. Flat irons also come in several materials such as ceramic, titanium and tourmaline. The ceramic flat irons heat more evenly on a consistent basis and they heat and cool relatively quickly.

Foundation – a cosmetic in liquid, cream, or cake form, usually colored, that is applied as a base for makeup.

Fungus – A fungal nail infection occurs when a fungus attacks a fingernail, a toenail, or the skin under the nail, called the nail bed. The most common symptom of a fungal nail infection is the nail becoming thickened and discolored.

Gel (Hair Gel) – a hairstyling product that is applied to wet hair and used to stiffen hair into a particular hairstyle, to aid in the styling process.

Gorgeous Woman – a woman battling cancer that is receiving or has received a full spa ambush-style makeover from Hello Gorgeous! or one of its Affiliate Salons!

Hair Spray – an aerosol or spritzing substance sprayed onto the hair to hold a hairstyle in place. Again, professional products found at prominent hair salons are always recommended over cheaper, retail store brands for the integrity of your hair.

Hair Substitution – any medium that takes the place of your hair during cancer treatment, for the purpose of warmth or concealment, such as a wig, hat, turban or scarf.

Hello Gorgeous! Affiliate Salon – an existing salon whose owner and team have the same passion to help women battling cancer with their appearance as does Hello Gorgeous! Among other duties, the salon must meet the criteria for acceptance; go through a three-hour training by a Hello Gorgeous! Affiliate coach; and perform a full spa, ambush-style makeover on a woman battling cancer in their community once a month.

Hello Gorgeous! of HOPE – our 501(c)(3) not-for-profit that provides a red-carpet experience for all women battling all cancers, with full spa ambush-style makeovers in one of our 36' mobile DaySpas or by one of our partnering Affiliate Salons across the United States. Each venue delivers spa services and cosmetic education in a salon environment, at no cost to these Gorgeous Women.

Highlight – common hair coloring process that is performed in a salon that involves foils or highlighting papers. This procedure can be done in full foils over the entirety of the head or with partial foils that only color some of the hair, for example, face-framing highlights.

Hot Rollers – plastic cylinders that your hair—or the hair on a human hair wig—can be wound around to produce curls in the hair. When heat is applied from a blow dryer, the hair retains some of the curl from the roller. Remember, synthetic wigs can never be heated without melting and ruining the wig.

Human-Hair Wig – a manufactured covering for the head made from harvested human hair. Human-hair wigs can be treated as real hair, and this includes washing, heat styling and coloring. Many human-hair wigs are available virgin, which is hair that has not been processed for color or texture and can therefore be customized to your liking. Human-hair wigs are also available in many colors, textures and curl patterns.

Lip Liner – a cosmetic, usually in soft pencil form, used to outline the lips before lipstick is applied.

Lipstick – an oily cosmetic in stick form, in a plastic or metal tube, used to color the lips.

Makeup Sponge – also called a cosmetic sponge, used to apply and remove certain types of makeup, moisturizer, and cleanser. They are available in many varieties and can be purchased at local drugstores and discount or high-end department stores. Depending on the purpose, they can be found in wedge shapes, round, puffs, infused with Vitamin E, smooth, rough, porous, dense, or any other shape or texture required to achieve the best application or removal of a product.

Manicure – a cosmetic treatment for the hands and nails that usually involves shaping and polishing the fingernails, pushing back the cuticles, and treating rough skin, performed at home or in a nail salon. During cancer treatment, it is important to take precautions both for extra sanitation and against any cuts or gouges to your hands or cuticles.

Mascara – eyelash cosmetic: thick colored paste applied to the eyelashes with a fine brush to darken them and give the appearance of greater length and thickness.

Moisturizer – also called emollients, are complex mixtures of chemical agents specially designed to make the external layers of the skin (epidermis)—especially the face—softer and more pliable. Facial moisturizers are recommended for women of all skin types and age groups to help skin retain moisture.

Mousse – hair mousse is a hair styling product that is dispensed in an aerosol foam spray. It adds volume to hair and often provides both conditioning and hold. Again, professional products found at hair salons are recommended over less expensive, retail store brands for the integrity of your hair.

Nail Clippers – a small pair of clippers used for trimming fingernails and toenails.

Nail Fast Dry – a clear liquid containing volatile silicones that causes the solvents in nail polish to evaporate quickly, thus drying the nail in seconds.

Nail Lifting – when a fingernail or toenail comes partially or fully detached from its nail bed due to a fungal infection, chemotherapy treatment, or some other type of trauma to the nail.

Nail Polish – a colored or transparent lacquer used to decorate fingernails or toenails.

Nippers – also called nail nippers or toenail nippers; used by professional Nail Technicians and podiatrists to trim cuticles and nails on feet and hands.

Non-Acetone Polish Remover – also a type of nail polish remover, it is generally made from ethyl acetate. Acetone-free nail polish removers are largely considered gentler for the nails and less likely to lead to excessive dryness and cracking.

On-The-Scalp Color – permanent or semi-permanent hair color, applied from your scalp to the ends of your hair follicles, to give your hair all-around color. This is the opposite of a highlight, which is applied to sections of your hair, with foils or highlight papers, in a broken pattern for emphasis.

Orangewood Stick – a thin stick, like a pencil, usually made of orangewood, with pointed and rounded ends used for cleaning fingernails and pushing back cuticles.

Over-the-Counter Cosmetic Products – Cosmetic products (hair, nail, skincare, color) not sold in a licensed, professional salon or supply house.

Many times sold in pharmacies, discount or grocery stores, OTC cosmetic products contain less expensive and inferior ingredients that usually cause the products to perform inadequately, compared to professional products.

Pastes (Hair Paste) – used to mold, control and shape your hair, allowing you to style your hair with amazing versatility and texture.

Patch Test – when a tiny portion or patch of a product is placed onto your skin to test for an allergic reaction. If you tend to be sensitive to any products at all, which can happen when going through chemotherapy, it is advisable to get your hairdresser to perform a patch test 48 hours before you have a color.

Pedicure – refers to superficial cosmetic treatment of the feet and toenails. A pedicure can help prevent nail diseases and nail disorders. Pedicures are done for cosmetic, therapeutic, and medical purposes; and are extremely popular throughout the world, primarily among women.

Pedicure Soak – a soap-based additive to pedicure baths that softens the cuticles and callused tissue of the feet.

Pedicure Scrub – a similar product to pedicure soak, usually containing an abrasive like pumice, used to soften feet in a foot bath before a pedicure.

Permanent Hair Color – a hair color designed to allow a single color to penetrate existing strands of hair, usually scalp to ends, and inject them with color that does not wash away. This color will eventually grow out, meaning that new growth must be dyed if uniform coloring is to be maintained.

Pomade – a greasy and waxy substance that is used to style hair. Pomade makes hair look slick, neat and shiny. Unlike hair spray and hair gel, pomade does not dry, and often takes several washes to remove. Again, professional products found at prominent hair salons are always recommended over cheaper, retail store brands for the integrity of your hair.

Powder – Powder makeup comes in either pressed or loose form. Pressed face powders are available in compacts that include a sponge or a powder puff for application purposes, while loose face powders come in a container with a sifter. Pressed eye shadows and blushes may be part of a palette of many colors or may be sold individually. Colored powder pigments can multitask as eye shadow, eyeliner, and blush.

Pumice Stone – a porous or spongy form of volcanic glass, used as an abrasive, and is an essential tool in giving a pedicure. It is used to remove dead skin and calluses from the feet.

Putty (Hair Putty) – Hair putty is a type of styling product that is usually thicker and sticky in consistency, a little stronger than gel or mousse. Putty usually makes the hairstyle stand up and have the very popular "messy" look. You can use it to separate sections of hair and make them go where you want.

Radiation Therapy – Radiation therapy, radiotherapy, or radiation oncology, often abbreviated RT, RTx, or XRT, is the medical use of ionizing radiation—generally as part of cancer treatment—to control or kill malignant cells.

Removable Bang – synthetic hair that is attached to a Velcro strip or connected to a headband, which can be worn easily under a turban, hat or scarf. The bangs can come in various widths. They can also range in lengths and colors.

Reveal – the term that Hello Gorgeous! of HOPE uses to represent the gathering of friends and family, usually in a public place like a restaurant, to witness the results of her ambush makeover.

Salon Products – Cosmetic products (hair, nail, skincare and color) sold exclusively in a licensed, professional salon or supply house. Salon products contain superior ingredients that allow the products to perform much better than an over-the-counter product.

Scarves – a large square of material used to create various coverings for your head, for warmth or to conceal hair loss. Four scarf-folding designs are included in this book, as well as in the video of scarf-tying on the included DVD.

Semi-Permanent Hair Color – hair dye that does not change the original color of the hair because semi-permanent hair color only deepens or lightens the natural hair color, without penetrating the entire hair shaft. This type of hair dye will not lighten hair but will change the hair a few shades or enhance the natural color. Most kinds of semi-permanent hair dye are made from organic material, including fruit extracts and henna.

Shampoo – a cleanser for the hair and scalp. Remember, professional products found at prominent hair salons are always recommended over less expensive, retail store brands for the integrity of your hair.

Spa Service – one of a number of cosmetic services, usually performed in a professional salon or day spa, such as a facial, manicure, pedicure, or massage.

Strand Test – where a small amount of the desired hair color is mixed up by your stylist, placed on a small section of your hair, and left there for the full processing time. The color is then removed with a towel and checked against the intended color, to make sure that you have achieved the desired results.

Synthetic Hair Wig – a manufactured covering for the head made of acrylic polymer strands resembling hair. They are available in many colors, textures and curl patterns. Because heat from styling tools can melt this material, many high-end synthetic wig manufacturers are beginning to use protein-based synthetic strands that more easily withstand direct exposure to high heat.

Toner – facial toners help to balance the pH level of your skin, tighten your facial pores (which allows fewer oils and toxins to settle into the skin), and help your skin to look brighter and healthier.

Top Coat – a clear coat that goes on last, over colored nail polish, and acts as a finishing coat. Top coats help to curb chipping of the nail paint and strengthen the entire manicure structure.

Turban – originally a head covering for men of Middle-Eastern descent, consisting of a long cloth wrapped in a pattern around their heads. Turbans for women are a one-piece covering of silk, cotton, or terrycloth and are worn many times during chemotherapy in the absence of hair.

Volumizing Product – Generally, there are three styling products that help create volume: Mousse foam, which should be applied to damp hair, starting at the roots and working down the hair's length; Volumizing spray, which is a lightweight product that adds body to hair; and Root-lifting products, sprayed directly on the roots of your hair only, providing lift and volume in the root area.

Wax (Hair Wax) – a thick hairstyling product containing wax, used to assist with holding the hair. It does not harden like products such as hair gel, but remains pliable.

Whiff Test – the simple act of smelling the wig cap area of a wig to see if it needs to be shampooed. A non-pleasant smell indicates it is time to wash the wig.

Wig Cap – the inside, rounded surface of a wig to which all the natural or synthetic hairs are attached, and that sits against your scalp while wearing the wig.

Wig Shampoo – a gentle shampoo specifically designed for synthetic wig cleaning.

Works Cited

– Abdullah, Ahmed, MD, FACS, FICS. "A History of Skincare and Cosmetics." Lexli.com. 3 March2014, 11 November, 2009. http://www.lexli.com/blog/archive/2009/11/11/a-history-of-skin-care-and-cosmetics.aspx

– Barrymore, John. "How to Match Colors to Your Skintone." HowStuffWorks.com. 5 March 2014. http://health.howstuffworks.com/skin-care/beauty/match-colors-to-your-skin-tone3.htm

– Brite, Kristine. "How to Apply Makeup For Hazel Eyes." Ehow.com/typef.com. 3 march, 2014. http://www.ehow.com/how_7664631_apply-eye-makeup-hazel-eyes.html

– Corbett-Owen, Cari. "People Need Touch to Thrive." Ditch Diets Live Light, 3 March, 2014. http://www.ditch-diets-live-light.com/massage-therapy-benefits.html

– Crutchfield III, Charles E. MD. "Dermatologists` Top 10 Tips for Relieving Dry Skin." Dermatology Nurse, 3 March, 2014. 1 October, 2006. http://www.webmd.com/beauty/dry-skin-13/cosmetic-procedures-skin-care-dry-skin

– Derrick, Julyne. "Lipstick Shades: How to Pick the Right One?" About.com. 3 March, 2014. http://beauty.about.com/od/plasticsurgery/qt/lip-color.htm

– Edwards, Christina. "What are the Different Types of Mascara?" Wisegeek, 3 March 2014. 14 April 2013. http://www.wisegeek.com/what-are-the-different-types-of-mascara.html

– Franks, Richard C. MD and Millar, Heather. "Your Hair After Chemo." WebMD.com. 3 March, 2014. 23 March 2012. http://blogs.webmd.com/cancer/2012/03/your-hair-after-chemo.html

– Freestone, Jennie. "Did You Know? – Importance of Skincare." Yahoo Voices, 3 March 2014. 13 October, 2010. http://voices.yahoo.com/did-know-importance-skin-care-6917008.html

– Gallagher, Lauren. "Good Hair On View In Ojikiere Show." 3 March, 2014. 7 July, 2013. http://www.sfexaminer.com/sanfrancisco/good-hair-on-view-in-ojeikere-show/Content?oid=2498545

- Gerson, Joel, Milady`s Standard Textbook for Professional Estheticians, 8th edition, pp. 14-20.
- Hamilton, David R. Ph.D. "Do Positive People Live Longer?" Huffington Post, 3 March 2014. 2 Nov, 2012. http://www.huffingtonpost.com/david-r-hamilton-phd/positive-people-live-long_b_774648.html
- Jochmann, Carmen. "Benefits of Human Touch." Suite 101, 3 March, 2014. 15 October, 2009. https://suite.io/carmen-jochmann/2ceq20k
- Jovanovic, Jelena. "8 Nail Shapes and How To Choose The Right One For You." Allwomentalk.com. 3 March, 2014 http://www.wisegeek.com/what-is-cosmetics-history.htm
- Madison, N. "Why do Women Wear Makeup?" Wisegeek, 3 March, 2014. 24 March , 2012. http://www.wisegeek.com/why-do-women-wear-makeup.html
- Marlena. "The Best Eyeshadow Color for Brown Eyes." Makeupgeek.com. 5 March, 2014. http://www.makeupgeek.com/articles/the-best-eyeshadow-colors-for-brown-eyes/
- Mojapelo, Charmaine. "It`s JUST Hair, Isn`t it?" DivasInc.com. 3 March, 2014. http://www.divasinc.co.za/2012/10/its-just-hair-isnt-it/
- Mayo Clinic Staff. "Chemotherapy and Hair Loss: What to Expect During Treatment." Mayo Clinic, 3 March, 2014. 6 March. 2012. http://www.mayoclinic.org/tests-procedures/chemotherapy/in-depth/hair-loss/art-20046920
- Nadine, Amy. "The Most Harmonious Blush Shade For Your Skintone." The Beauty Department, 3 March, 2014. August 2010. http://www.thebeautydepartment.com/2012/08/the-most-harmonious-blush-shade-for-your-skin-tone/
- Page, Danielle. "5 Reasons Not to Wear Makeup to Bed." TheExaminer.com. 5 March 2014, 6 May, 2009. http://www.examiner.com/article/top-5-reasons-not-to-sleep-with-your-makeup-on
- Peterson, Erica. "What is Cosmetics' History?" Wisegeek.com. 5 March 2014. http://www.wisegeek.com/what-is-cosmetics-history.htm
- Rogers, Cathy. Why did Women Start Painting Their Nails?" Wisegeek, 3 March, 2014. 17 February, 2014. http://www.wisegeek.com/when-did-women-start-painting-their-nails.html
- Rouleau, Renee. "11 Common Causes for Acne and Blemishes." Renee Rouleau.com. 3 March, 2014. 8 June, 2010. http://www.examiner.com/article/top-5-reasons-not-to-sleep-with-your-makeup-on Seagal, Jeanne Ph.D and Smith, Melinda, M.A. "Laughter is the Best Medicine". Helpguide.org, 5 March 2014, 4 April, 2013.
- Scheve, Tom. "What Would Happen if You Never Moisturized Your Face?" Discovery Health, 3 March, 2014. September, 2012. http://health.howstuffworks.com/skin-care/moisturizing/basics/never-moistur-

ized-face.html "Wig", Wikipedia, 3 March, 2014. July, 2009. http://en.wikipedia.org/wiki/Wig

– Segal, Jeanne Ph.D and Smith, Melinda MA. "Laughter is The Best Medicine." HelpGuide.org. 3 March, 2014. http://www.helpguide.org/life/humor_laughter_health.htm

– Shabana, Mir. "17 Reasons Why Women Wear Headscarves." USC Annenberg, 3 March, 2014. 27 March. 2008. http://www.religiondispatches.org/archive/sexandgender/152/17_reasons_why_women_wear_headscarves

– Stibich, Mark Ph.D. "10 Reasons to Smile". About.com/Healthy Aging, 3 March 2014, 22 Jan 2013. http://longevity.about.com/od/lifelongbeauty/tp/smiling.htm

– Walton, Tracey. "Is Massage Safe for People Living With Cancer?" TraceyWalton.com. 5 March, 2014. http://tracywalton.com/faqs/index.html

– "20 Gorgeous Makeup Ideas for Green Eyes." 3 March 2014. http://www.stylemotivation.com/20-gorgeous-makeup-ideas-for-green-eyes/

– Good News Bible. Susan Lightly, ed. Birmingham: Liturgical Publications, 1954.

– "Guide to Styling Your Body Shape." Ask.com/Thechickfashionistas/bodyshapes. 3 march, 2014. http://www.thechicfashionista.com/body-shapes.html

– "Hat Wearing Guide for Cancer Therapy Patients." Headcovers.com. 3 March, 2014. http://www.headcovers.com/hats.php

– "History of Cosmetics." Wikipedia.com. 3 March 2014. http://en.wikipedia.org/wiki/History_of_cosmetics

– "History of Wigs." E-Wigs, 3 March 2014. http://www.e-wigs.com./history-of-wigs.html

– "How to Choose the Right Mascara." Squidoo.com. 3 March, 2014. http://betsuzie.squidoo.com/mascarareviews

– "Fashion." Wikipedia.com. 3 March 2014.
   http://en.wikipedia.org/fashion

– "How To Dress Your Body Type". Shop Your Shape.com, 3 March, 2014. 10 April. 2014. http://www.shopyourshape.com/body-shapes.html

– "Pedicures." Wikipedia.com. 3 March, 2014. http://en.wikipedia.org/wiki/Pedicure

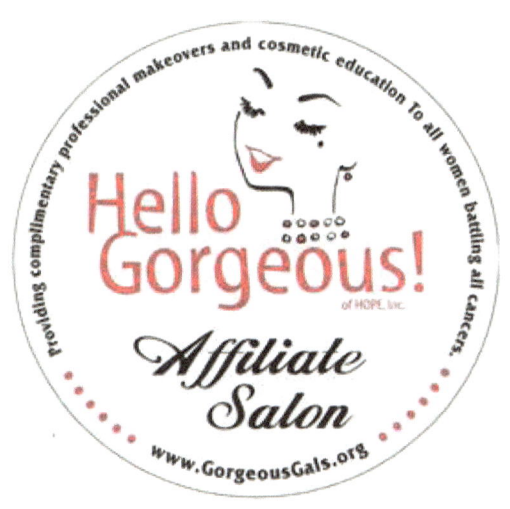

Current List of Our Affiliate Salons

CALIFORNIA
Headlines, the Salon, Encinitas, CA

FLORIDA
Bonita Springs School, Bonita Springs, FL
Oasis Salon and Spa, Bonita Springs, FL

ILLINOIS
Aqua Salon, Chicago, IL
Studio One Salon and Spa, Gurnee, IL

INDIANA
A Plus Hair Studio, Crown Point, IN
Bangs Salon and Spa, South Bend, IN

The Beauty Shoppe, Elkhart, IN
The Beehive, South Bend, IN
CC Hair Company, Plymouth, IN
Chateau Bijou, Noblesville, IN
Creative Edge Hair Studio , Mishawaka, IN
Expressions Day Spa, Warsaw, IN
Express Yourself Salon and Day Spa, Elkhart
FIX Spa Salon, Elkhart, IN
LeRoc Salon and Body Bar, Valparaiso, IN
Michelle's Headquarters, Culver, IN
Nicholas J Salon and Spa, Notre Dame, IN
Sandy's Hair Design, South Bend, IN
Solutions Salon and Day Spa, Kokomo, IN
Vintage Coco, Granger, IN

IOWA
Blush Salon and Spa, Cedar Rapids

MARYLAND
NUVO Salon and Spa, Frederick, MD
Studio She, Frederick MD

MICHIGAN
Seasons of Hair Salon, Holland, MI
Studio 1, Saint Joseph, MI

MINNESOTA
Aspasia Salon and Spa, Saint Charles, MN
New Reflections Salon and Day Spa, Plymouth, MN

PENNSYLVANIA
Alternative Spa and Salon, Corry, PA

Scan this QR Code for Apple or Android phones

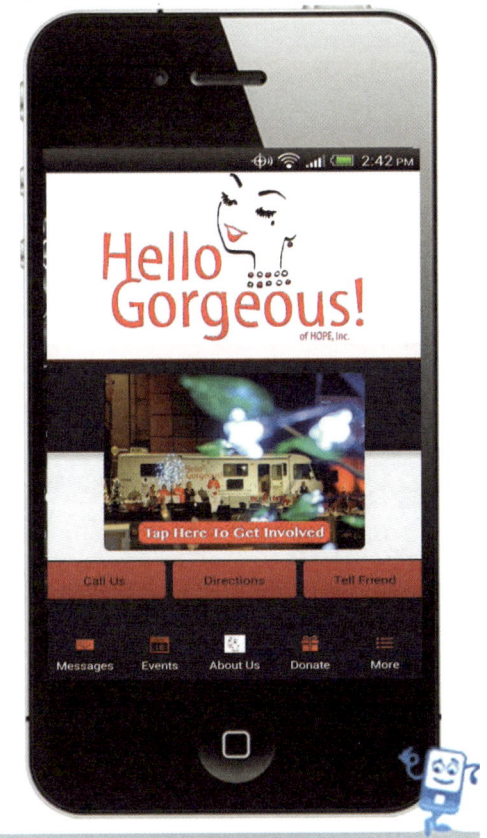

or
Stay connected with Hello Gorgeous!

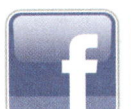 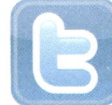